# MACROBIOTIC
# WELLNESS

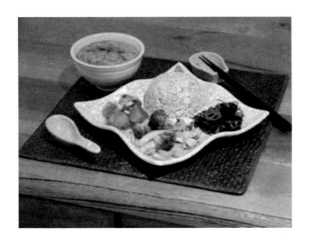

*Plant-Based Dietary Guidelines*
*For Health & Vitality*

Alex Jack, Bettina Zumdick
Edward Esko

Planetary Health, Inc.

Macrobiotic Wellness
By Alex Jack, Bettina Zumdick, and Edward Esko

© 2020 by Planetary Health, Inc.

ISBN: 9781548158798


Published by Amberwaves Press
PO Box 487, Becket MA 01223
413-623-0012

www.macrobioticsummerconference.com
www.amberwavesofgrain.com
www.makropedia.com
www.ebolaanddiet.com

Printed in the U.S.A.

First edition 2020

# Hippocratic Oath Pledges to Use Culinary Medicine

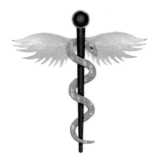

*The Hippocratic Oath, composed by Hippocrates, the Father of Medicine, 2500 years ago, pledges to apply "dietetic measures for the benefit of the sick." Modern medicine replaced the culinary approach of the original Greek with "do no harm," since modern medicine no longer focuses on diet and nutrition. The original Oath also prohibits the use of deadly drugs, surgery, and other practices that govern healthcare today and which are often unnecessary or harmful:*

I swear by Apollo Physician and Asclepius and Hygieia and Panacea and all the gods and goddesses, making them my witnesses, that I will fulfill according to my ability and judgment this oath and this covenant:

To hold him who has taught me this art as equal to my parents and to live my life in partnership with him . . .

**I will apply dietetic measures for the benefit of the sick according to my ability and judgment: I will keep them from harm and injustice.**

I will neither give a deadly drug to anybody if asked for it, nor will I make a suggestion to this effect. Similarly, I will not give to a woman an abortive remedy. In purity and holiness, I will guard my life and my art.

I will not use the knife, not even on sufferers from stone, but will withdraw in favor of such men as are engaged in this work.

Whatever houses I may visit, I will come for the benefit of the sick, remaining free of all intentional injustice, of all mischief, and in particular of sexual relations with both female and male persons, be they free or slaves.

What I may see or hear in the course of the treatment or even outside of the treatment in regard to the life of men, which on no account one must spread abroad, I will keep to myself holding such things shameful to be spoken about.

If I fulfill this oath and do not violate it, may it be granted to me to enjoy life and art, being honored with fame among all men for all time to come; if I transgress it and swear falsely, may the opposite of all this be my lot.

*The translation is from the original Greek in* Ancient Medicine: Selected Papers of Ludwig Edelstein, *translated by Owsei Temkin and C. Lilian Temkin (Johns Hopkins University Press, 1961).*

# Preface

"Let food be thy medicine, and thy medicine be food."—Hippocrates

During the last half century, modern macrobiotics has been in the forefront of the health and diet revolution, serving as the catalyst for many of the dietary and lifestyle changes now circling the globe. Macrobiotics has introduced modern societies to organically grown whole foods and naturally processed foods, including brown rice, whole wheat, and other whole grains; miso, tofu, tempeh, and other traditional soy products; a cornucopia of fresh garden vegetables; wakame, kombu, and other sea vegetables; and a variety of high-quality seasonings, condiments, and sugar- and dairy-free desserts and snacks. Macrobiotics has also popularized holistic health, self-healing, and alternative and complementary methods that are now embraced by millions of people and by the medical profession.

"Macrobiotics" comes from *makrobios*, the Greek term for "Long Life" and "Great Life." Hippocrates, the Father of Medicine, coined the word, and in the modern era it has been developed by Michio and Aveline Kushi and other educators in North America, South America, Europe, Asia, Africa, and the Middle East. By creating our minds and bodies from whole natural foods in a spirit of thankfulness, we can contribute to personal health, social well-being, and planetary health and peace.

The benefits of a macrobiotic diet are widely recognized today, as the scientific and medical studies and other accounts in this book show. From a tiny seed in the 1960s, macrobiotic principles have blossomed into a tree of life, nourishing society at many levels. The landmark dietary and nutritional changes over the last generation have been influenced and shaped by macrobiotics, from *Dietary Goals for the United States,* the landmark report by a Select U.S. Senate Committee in the late 1970s, to the government's Food Guide Pyramid in the 1980s, from the creation of the Office of Alternative Medicine within the National Institutes of Health (NIH) in the 1990s to the shift toward a plant-centered diet and vegan cuisine in the 2000s.

The momentous changes that took place constitute a nutritional axis shift. The Basic Four food groups—based on meat and dairy food—were replaced with a more balanced way of eating centered on grains, vegetables, fruits, and other plant foods. As the new century began, the *U.S. Dietary Guidelines* accompanying the Food Guide Pyramid called upon Americans to "use plant foods as the foundation of your meals":

There are many ways to create a healthy eating pattern, but they all start with the three food groups at the base of the Pyramid: grains, fruits, and vegetables. Eating a variety of grains (especially whole grain foods), fruits, and vegetables is the basis of healthy eating. Enjoy meals that have rice, pasta, tortillas, or whole grain bread as the center of the plate. . . . Eating plenty of whole grains, such as whole grain bread or oatmeal, as part of the healthful eating patterns described by these guidelines, may help protect you against many chronic diseases.[1]

The benefits of a macrobiotic way of eating have been recognized by the major scientific and medical societies and published in leading journals, including the *New England Journal of Medicine, Journal of the American Medical Association, American Journal of Clinical Nutrition, Lancet*, and many others.

Over the years, we have cooperated with many researchers and medical institutions. This year, through Planetary Health, Inc., we are planning to conduct our own study—a whole foods dietary intervention trial for people with Type 2 diabetes—under the auspices of the Berkshire Medical Center, a large hospital in western Massachusetts. We are hopeful that this little book will be beneficial for patients and families who will be enrolled in this study as well as others who are beginning the macrobiotic way of life.

We are also making this material available because the Trump Administration this past year jettisoned the time-honored scientific process of determining national dietary guidelines and announced that all research studies prior to 2000 were obsolete and would not be considered. These include scores of macrobiotic nutritional and medical studies published in leading medical journals over the last generation. These peer-reviewed papers were instrumental in developing the Food Guide Pyramid, MyPlate, and other dietary guidelines for Americans. Instead of impartial and open-minded scientists, the White House entrusted responsibility for the 2020 national guidelines to a panel composed of specialists with ties to the beef, dairy, and soft drink industries.

Amnesia and special interests are poor qualifications for formulating policy on public health and planetary destiny, especially since diet is a leading cause of global warming and climate change. We are summarizing these important studies in this book so that they will not be forgotten and be available for future nutritionists, physicians, and researchers. The abuse of history and scientific truth is all the more reason to launch new, fresh studies. We welcome your support in this effort. Together we can create a world of enduring health, happiness, and peace.

Alex Jack, Bettina Zumdick, and Edward Esko
The Berkshires
November 2019

# Contents

Hippocratic Oath  3
Preface  4
Macrobiotics  7
7 Qualities of Balanced Food  8
5 Key Elements  10
Avoiding Ultra-processed food  12
Standard Macrobiotic Dietary
  Guidelines  14
Way of Eating Suggestions  18
Kitchenware  18
Lifestyle Guidelines  19
Progressive Development of Disease
  20
The Spiral of Natural Healing  22
Food as Medicine  24
Scientific and Medical Studies  27
  The 1st Nutritional Experiment  27
  Macrobiotics & Whole Food
    Nutrition 28
  Heart Disease  31
  Cancer  33
    Breast  37
    Colon  39
    Endometrial  40
    Lung  41
    Pancreatic  41
    Prostate  42
    Stomach  43
  General Medical Opinion  43
  AIDS  45
  Arthritis  47
  Autism  48
  Celiac Disease  49
  Children's Health  50
  Crohn's Disease  51
  Diabetes 52
  Ebola  53

Environmental Illness  54
Geriatric 55
Gluten Intolerance  55
Hospital Food  56
Medical Education  57
Mental and Emotional Health  58
Microwave Cooking  59
Migraine and PMS  59
Multiple Sclerosis  60
Nuclear Radiation  60
Obesity  62
Osteoporosis  63
Pregnancy and Childcare  63
Lifestyle  66
  Chewing  66
  Exercise and Fitness  66
  Arts and Culture  67
Social Health  68
  Ancient Food Pattern  68
  Agriculture & GMOs  71
  Crime and Violence  72
  Peace and Social Justice  74
Planetary Health  77
  Nutrient Decline  77
  Global Warming  77
  Electromagnetic Fields  79
  Energy and Transmutation 80
  Light Pollution  82
The Coming Era  83
Daily Menus & Recipes  84
Home Remedies  90
Supplements 92
Regional Guidelines  93
2020 U.S. Dietary Guidelines  98
Glossary  101
Macrobiotic Resources  107
References  111

*Symbols used in this book*

🌾 Macrobiotic case histories, reports, articles (sheaf of grain)

⚕ Scientific or medical studies, reports, articles (caduceus healing wand)

# Macrobiotics

Macrobiotics is the art of living a bright, healthy, peaceful life. It encompasses a deep understanding of humanity's origin and destiny, natural order, and the cosmos. It encompasses evolution and history, climate and environment, anatomy and physiology, behavior and activity, thoughts and emotions, relationships and communities, arts and cultures, science and medicine, societies and civilizations, and consciousness and spiritual development.

A macrobiotic diet and lifestyle is grounded in a way of eating centered on whole grains and other primarily plant-based foods and on living in harmony and balance with nature and the infinite universe. It embraces all complementary opposites, including East and West, North and South, traditional and modern, material and spiritual, visionary and practical, and strives to create a peaceful mind, home, and world community.[2]

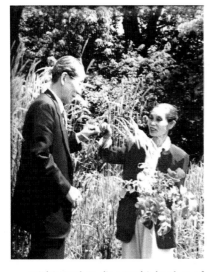

**Michio and Aveline Kushi, leaders of the modern macrobiotic movement.**

The macrobiotic movement, led by educators Michio Kushi (1926-2014) and his wife Aveline Kushi (1926-2001), pioneered the natural foods movement, organic farming, and alternative healing beginning in the 1960s and over the last half century spearheaded the historical shift in modern society from an animal- to a plant-based diet.[3] During this time, macrobiotics has been studied by the National Institutes of Health (NIH), CDC (Center for Disease Control and Prevention), Harvard Medical School, Framingham Heart Study, and other scientific and medical organizations.[4]

Its positive benefits in helping to prevent and relieve high blood pressure, high cholesterol, and heart disease; selected cancers, diabetes; immune-deficiency dis-eases; and other chronic conditions have been published in the *New England Journal of Medicine, American Journal of Clinical Nutrition, Lancet, Nutrition and Cancer,* and other peer-reviewed journals. As *The American Medical Association Family Medical Guide* concluded: "In general, the macrobiotic diet is a healthful way of eating."[5]

The Smithsonian Institution recognized the contribution of macrobiotics to "healthy diet, our increasingly global culture, alternative healing, peace studies, and traditions of grassroots activism" with the creation of a permanent Michio and Aveline Kushi Collection at the National Museum of American History in Washington, D.C. in 1998.[6] The macrobiotic community today continues to be on the cutting edge of personal and planetary change with a global network of thousands of teachers, counselors, and chefs, as well as educational centers, communities, organic farms, natural foods companies, restaurants, businesses, small publishers, and social media.

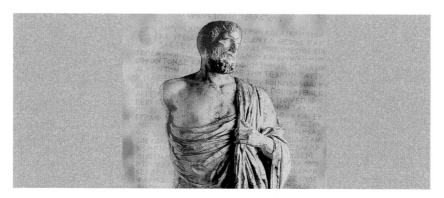

*Hippocrates, the Father of Medicine, coined the term* macrobios *(long life) about 2500 years ago.*

# 7 Qualities of Balanced Food

**1. Whole** means whole, natural or unrefined food; for example, brown rice is preferred to white rice and whole wheat to white flour. Whole natural food retains the full energy (*Ki, Chi,* or Prana) of the food after harvest and is ideal for optimal daily health and vitality. Whole food is also higher in nutrients, antioxidants, phytoestrogens, and other health-giving compounds. For example, whole-grain rice and whole wheat retain from 50 to 100 percent more complex carbohydrates, fiber, vitamins, minerals, and trace elements than refined grains.

**2. Organic** foods are grown without chemical fertilizers, herbicides, pesticides, or other artificial sprays. Nor do they contain preservatives, colorings, or other artificial ingredients, including GMOs, growth hormones, and vaccines.

**3. Seasonal** signifies that we eat perishable foods in the season they are grown, harvested, or stored. For example, fresh fruits retain optimal energy in late spring, summer, or early fall; sprouts, radishes, cucumbers, and other garden veggies in spring and summer; squashes and pumpkins in fall and winter; and grains, beans, root vegetables, and sea vegetables keep well throughout the year.

**4. Ecological** eating respects the climate and environment in which foods are grown. For example, in the United States, which is mostly a four-season climate, the more healthful fruits to eat are apples, pears, peaches, berries, melons, and other temperate fruits rather than pineapples, mangoes, and other tropical fare. (These larger, juicier fruits, however, are suitable in warmer latitudes.) Practically speaking, foods that grow in an east or west direction from where we live are suitable for regular use, including produce from California if we live on the East Coast or from Europe, Russia, China, Japan, and other places that share a similar climate. Eating foods that grow significantly north or south from where we live violates natural climactic and environmental boundaries and may lead to imbalances and an inability to adapt to our surroundings. Hence, in temperate regions we avoid or minimize hot spices (from the tropics) or heavy meat and dairy foods (from the cold North, high mountains, or desert regions). However, in their native locales, these can be considered part of a traditional way of eating.

**5. Naturally processed foods** or unprocessed foods are stronger and more vitalizing than processed foods. For example, whole oats give strong, warming energy, while Irish or steel-cut oats that have been mechanically cut into quarters or smaller pieces retain less *Ki* or vital energy and are not as hardy, as their strong, whole energy begins to disperse. Scottish oats, rolled oats, or oat flakes that have been further reduced and cook up even more quickly than Irish oats contain the least amount of energy and vitality. All types of oats may be part of a balanced way of eating. For the most part, a majority of our grains and other foods should be in whole form and a smaller portion naturally processed.

Naturally processed foods also include tofu, tempeh, miso, shoyu, and other traditionally made soy foods, as well as pickles, natural sweeteners, condiments, seasonings, and beverages that have been fermented or traditionally or minimally processed. These foods are an important part of the macrobiotic way of eating as long as they are made from the highest quality ingredients, aged naturally, and avoid high temperatures, pressures, and other artificial or extreme processing methods. They give a totally different energy than textured soy protein, soy meat substitutes, and other highly processed foods. The use of condiments, seasonings, and garnishes is an easy way to modify tastes and flavors.

**6. Locally grown** foods that grow in our own area are generally fresher and more balanced than those that originate from across the country or around the globe. They also require less transportation, packaging, and distribution and are gentler on the earth. Growing your own food in a backyard organic garden is ideal. Next best is obtaining locally grown food from farmers' markets or CSA—Community Supported Agriculture—or purchasing shares of produce from local farms.

**7. Sustainable** foods benefit the planet as a whole, including the water, the air, the valleys and mountains, the plants, and human beings and other animals. Besides cattle plantations, giant agribusiness companies today are producing organic soybeans, maize, palm oil, and other monocultures that are threatening rainforests in South America, Southeast Asia, and elsewhere and are contributing to global warming and the loss of diversity. Similarly, the demand for quinoa, the traditional grain of the ancient Incans, in modern society has driven up prices and made it unaffordable to native Peruvians and Bolivians. Such foods are unsustainable. Fortunately, quinoa is now being grown in California, Colorado, and other regions and can be used instead of the Andean variety.

## Five Key Elements

When properly cooked or prepared, balanced foods share five further qualities. They are fresh, tasty and delicious, beautiful, balanced, and full of *Ki*.

**1. Fresh** food includes grains, beans, veggies, fruits, seeds, and nuts just harvested from the garden or brought to market, or naturally processed products such as tofu and tempeh freshly made at home or purchased as soon as available. In a balanced, plant-based kitchen, industrially mass-produced foods, such as instant foods, canned foods, frozen foods, refined grains and flour, sprayed foods, dyed foods, irradiated foods, genetically engineered foods, and chemically grown or treated foods are avoided.

**2. Tasty and delicious** is a phrase foreign to many health foods. On the contrary, health foods have a reputation for being bland and tasteless. Macrobiotic cooking is widely appreciated for its exquisite flavor, taste, and texture. Because macrobiotics is based on principles of balance and harmony, food prepared this way quenches the appetite, delights the palate, and leaves one with a feeling of deep satisfaction and contentment. Of course, the art of macrobiotic cooking takes time to learn and master. But whether you are a beginner or an experienced chef, you will soon start preparing food that the entire family, friends, and colleagues will truly enjoy.

**3. Beautiful** food adds another layer of sensory enjoyment, aesthetic satisfaction, and spiritual serenity to the meal. The art of plating strives to make each dish or meal an artistic masterpiece. Garnishes, sauces and dressings, icings, and other special toppings, fillings, and touches enhance the beauty of the meal. Special plates, bowls, serving dishes, utensils, napkins, and other cookware featuring natural colors and textures further accentuate the dining experience. Finally, flowers, leaves, pinecones, gourds, seashells, or other seasonal flourishes at the table make the meal a memorable experience.

**4. Balanced** food consciously blends principles of balance and harmony to create a meal that is greater than the sum of its parts. Ideally, each meal is based on our planet's biological evolution and humanity's traditional way of eating, the climate and environment, the season and weather, sex and age, and the personal health, vitality, and needs of everyone at the table. For example, at the start of a meal, miso, a fermented soybean product with living enzymes, is frequently used to make soup that replicates the ancient ocean in which primitive life began. Today, wild grains and grasses, the traditional staples of humanity, are consumed largely in the form of cultivated whole grains, noodles and pasta, and other grain products such as bread, seitan, and fu. Sea vegetables offer a subtle, unique energy from the ancient sea that balances vegetables, fruits, seeds and nuts, and more recent plant life that evolved on land. By consuming foods from land and sea, mountain and plain, above and below ground, we take in the entire spiral of life on our planet and develop a comprehensive mind and universal spirit.

**5. Radiating Life energy** (*Ki*) flows naturally between heaven and earth. All living things radiate natural electromagnetic energy. This energy is especially concentrated in seeds. Whole unhulled rice, for example, naturally retains its *Ki* energy for years—centuries and millennia, in some cases—and like other whole cereal grains is a principal food for longevity. Beans, seeds and nuts, and sea vegetables also retain their vitality over time. Ancient lotus root seeds dating to fifteen hundred years ago recently propagated and gave birth to strong, healthy new offspring. Of course, a balanced macrobiotic meal might also include leafy greens, delicate soups, quick crispy vegetables, fresh fruit, and other lighter, more perishable fare to balance the strong life force in the hardy grains, beans, and other seeds that are the foundation of a long, happy life.

Ki energy can be further enhanced through special farming and gardening techniques, cooking methods, artfully designed cookware, serene music, and grace at meals, prayer, meditation, chanting, and other spiritual practices. Unfortunately, most modern food, especially fast food and artificial food, is dead, dying, or depleted and has little or no ki. As a result, the nutrients in food have steadily declined in recent decades. The use of new high-yielding hybrid seeds and marketing methods that emphasize shelf life over freshness have weakened most industrially grown and artificially processed food. As much as possible, foods should be made with heirloom, open-pollinated, standard, or nonhybrid seeds that retain the life force and vitality of the original variety.

Food with Ki energy radiates life, peace, and harmony. Dead food, dying food, or food with excessively high or low energy includes food grown with chemical fertilizers, pesticides, and other sprays; factory-farmed meat, poultry, eggs, and dairy; farm-raised fish; and other mass-produced animal food; most canned, bottled, and frozen foods (unless traditionally processed); foods containing additives, preservatives, colors, flavorings, and other artificial ingredients; irradiated food; and genetically modified food. These foods are not alive.

**Awned grains** in particular are recommended. Awns are the long bristles on the heads of growing grains. Like antennae, they absorb the higher energies and vibrations of the cosmos and heighten our consciousness when we eat them. For the most part, whole barley and whole wheat (and their products) are awned and highly recommended for regular use. For the most part, rice is not awned. Unlike barley and wheat, awned rice is much harder to harvest than awnless varieties and gives reduced yields. Historically, awnless rice was preferred, and today most rice, whether brown or white, is awnless. A small volume of awned rice is now being grown and used primarily for ceremonial use. We hope it will become more widely available for regular use. For culinary medicinal purposes, awnless rice is still very beneficial and recommended.

## Avoid Ultra-Processed Food

Modern nutrition continues to evolve. In the early and mid 20th century, it focused on identifying sources of adequate calories and essential vitamins, minerals, and other ingredients often missing in the diet. This approach helped prevent scurvy, beriberi, and nutritional deficiency diseases, but it failed to stem the epidemic of heart disease, cancer, diabetes, and other chronic illnesses caused by the intake of excessive nutrients. *More* in the standard American diet turned out to be *less*.

Beginning in the 1960s and 1970s, the natural foods and whole foods movements helped rectify this oversight by focusing on whole vs. processed food and by taking into account whether food was grown organically, chemically, or with genetic engineering. As Dr. Colin Campbell, the director of the China Study, the world's largest epidemiological study concluded in the 1990s and early 2000s on the basis of actual disease and death rates, there is a fundamental difference between plant-based and animal-based protein and other nutrients.

Plant or green protein from grains, beans, tofu, and other vegetal sources is metabolized differently from meat and dairy protein and does not contribute to the leading degenerative diseases of modern society. For example, the Chinese who traditionally consume almost no dairy products, have very low osteoporosis rates, while Americans who eat large amounts of calcium-rich milk, cheese, and other dairy foods have a high incidence of this bone-thinning disease. As a result of studies like this, the U.S. government replaced the Four Food Groups, centered on animal foods, with the Food Guide Pyramid focusing on whole grains, fresh fruits and vegetables, and other plant foods as the foundation of a healthy, balanced daily food pattern.

The trend toward a plant-based diet in the early 21st century has improved the health of millions of people and benefited society at many levels. Coronary heart disease rates have fallen sharply, cancer has peaked, and other chronic diseases linked to animal protein and hard saturated fat have fallen. However, this approach still does not go far enough. Many vegetarians, vegans, and flexitarians (who eat mostly plant-based foods but occasional animal foods) still get diabetes, asthma, and breast cancer, even though they have substantially reduced or given up meat and dairy.

The problem is not all plant-based foods are created equal. There is a world of difference between a home-cooked meal with food fresh from the garden or farmers' market and factory farmed meat or industrially produced fake meats and vegan pre-prepared foods. Today, 58% of the food consumed in America comes from prepared convenience foods, including mass-produced burgers and pizza (both meat- and plant-based), instant soups, and milks (both dairy and non-dairy).

To help address the wave of ultra-processed food, the latest trend in nutrition science is to use a classification system that separates food, including plant-rich food, into categories based on how processed the food is. The most common is the NOVA Food classification System developed by scientists at the University of Sao Paulo in Brazil. The firve categories and samples include:

1. **Unprocessed**: brown rice, whole wheat, whole barley, and other whole grains; chickpeas, lentils, and other beans and legumes; fresh fruits and vegetables; sea vegetables; seeds and nuts and other foods that are intact

2. **Minimally processed**: natural foods with inedible or unwanted parts removed and lightly boiled, fermented crushed, ground, filtered, frozen, or chilled. Samples include tofu, tempeh, and other traditionally processed bean products; oatmeal; pre-cut produce; sesame, olive, and other unrefined oils; frozen fruits and vegetables; and pasteurized food

3. **Processed culinary ingredients**: substances from Group 1 that involve pressing, grinding, milling, drying, or refining and may include added sugar, salt, butter, or plant oils

4. **Processed foods**: foods that are industrially preserved, prepared, or cooked, including canned, bottled, salted, sugared, or cured foods, including beer, cider, and wine.

5. **Ultra-processed foods**: mass processed foods with typically five or more ingredients, including ingredients extracted from foods such as casein, lactose, whey, and gluten and some derived from further processing of food components, including hydrogenated oils, hydrolyzed proteins, soy protein isolate, maltodextrin, invert sugar, and high fructose corn syrup. Such products may also include dyes, color stabilizers, flavors enhancers, and processing aids such as carbonating, firming, bulking, and anti-bulking agents, emulsifiers, and humectants. Examples include carbonated drinks, sweet or savory packaged snacks, ice cream, candies, mass-produced breads and buns, margarines and spreads, cookies, pastries, cakes, breakfast cereals, energy bars, energy drinks, infant formulas, soy and other plant-based milks, and vegan burgers, hot dogs, sausages, cheeses, and other mock meats.

For optimal health and wellness, daily fare should include foods primarily from Group 1 and occasionally (up to several times a week) from Group 2. Processed foods and ultra-processed foods in Groups 3 and 4 should be avoided or consumed irregularly (several times a month or less), primarily on social occasions or for enjoyment. Processed and ultra-processed foods may be regarded as party foods for special occasions or, in a pinch, while traveling, though delicious, healthful festive foods and travel foods can easily be made from scratch with whole unprocessed and minimally processed ingredients. For those who are healing, it is essential to consume unprocessed and minimally processed foods and strictly avoid processed and ultra-processed items until usual good health has been restored.

# Standard Dietary & Way of Life Suggestions
*For persons living in a temperate climate*

## Daily Dietary Recommendations

**WHOLE CEREAL GRAINS** From 40–50% by weight of daily food includes cooked, organically grown, whole cereal grains prepared in a variety of ways. Whole cereal grains include brown rice, barley, millet, whole wheat, rye, oats, corn, and buckwheat. A portion of this amount may consist of noodles or pasta, unyeasted whole grain breads, and other partially processed whole cereal grains.

**SOUPS** About 5–10% of your daily food intake may include soup made with vegetables, sea vegetables (especially wakame or kombu), grains, or beans. Seasonings are usually miso or shoyu (organic soy sauce). The flavor should be moderate.

**VEGETABLES** About 25–30% of daily intake may include local and organically grown vegetables. The majority are preferably cooked in various styles (e.g., sautéed with a small amount of vegetable oil, steamed, boiled, and sometimes as raw salad or naturally fermented or pickled vegetables). Vegetables for daily use include green cabbage, kale, broccoli, cauliflower, collards, pumpkin, watercress, Chinese cabbage, bok choy, mustard greens, daikon greens, scallion, onion, daikon, turnip, various fall and winter season squashes, burdock, carrot, and onion. Lettuce, summer squash, cucumber, sprouts and other seasonal vegetables may be used less often. Avoid or limit the intake of white potato, sweet potato and yam, tomato, eggplant, pepper, spinach, asparagus, beets, zucchini, and avocado. Mayonnaise and other oily, fatty, or artificial dressings, including most commercial vegan spreads, are best avoided.

**BEANS AND SEA VEGETABLES** About 5–10% of the daily diet may include cooked beans and sea vegetables. Beans for regular use include azuki, chickpea, lentil, and black soybean, as well as kidney, navy, black bean, white bean, pinto, non-GMO soybean, and others. Bean products such as tofu, tempeh, and natto can also be used. Sea vegetables such as wakame, nori, kombu, hiziki, arame, dulse, agar, and others may be prepared in a variety of ways. They can be cooked with beans or vegetables, used in soups, or served separately as side dishes or salads, moderately flavored with brown rice vinegar, sea salt, shoyu, ume plum, and other natural seasonings.

**OCCASIONAL FOODS**
Fruit or fruit desserts including fresh, dried, and cooked fruits, may also be served 3–4 times per week. Local and organically grown fruits are preferred. If you live in a temperate climate, avoid tropical and semi-tropical fruit and instead enjoy apples, pears, plums, peaches, nectarines, apricots, berries, and melons. Locally organic fruit juice and cider may also be taken if your condition permits.

Lightly roasted nuts and seeds such as pumpkin, sesame, and sunflower may be enjoyed as snacks along with peanuts, walnuts, almonds, and pecans. Rice syrup, barley malt, amasake, and mirin may be used as sweeteners, together with maple syrup on special occasions. Brown rice vinegar, lemon, or umeboshi vinegar may be used for a sour taste.

**BEVERAGES** Recommened daily beverages include bancha twig tea (kucicha), stem tea roasted brown rice, roasted barley tea, and occasionally dandelion and corn silk tea. Any traditional tea that does not have an aromatic fragrance or a stimulating effect can be used. You may also drink a comfortable amount of water, preferably spring or well water (though filtered is acceptable), but avoid icy, cold drinks.

**ANIMAL FOOD** Animal food is not needed for daily health and vitality, and a balanced vegan diet is ideal. For those who choose to eat animal food for stronger energy, in transition from a conventional meat-based diet, or for medicinal purposes, a small volume of fish or seafood (once or twice a week) is preferable to meat or poultry. White-meat fish such as cod, haddock, and sole are less fatty, less oily, and more healthful than tuna, salmon, shrimp, and other red-meat and blue-skin varieties. In a world of polluted oceans and rapid climate change, the less fish and seafood consumed the better for personal and planetary health.

**FOODS TO REDUCE OR AVOID** For better health and well-being, limit or discontinue meat, animal fat and protein, eggs, poultry, dairy products (including butter, yogurt, ice cream, milk, and cheese), refined sugars, chocolate, molasses, honey, and other simple sugars such as stevia, agave, evaporated cane juice, and foods containing them.

- Tropical or semi-tropical fruits and fruit juices, including banana, pine-apple, mango, and papaya, as well as soda, cola, artificial drinks and beverages, coffee, decaf, colored tea, and all aromatic stimulating teach such as mint or peppermint.

- All refined and polished grains, flours, and their derivatives. Mass-produced industrialized food, including canned, frozen, and irradiated food.

- All artificially colored, preserved, sprayed or chemically treated foods, including foods with GMOs.

- Hot spices, any aromatic, stimulating food or food accessory, artificial vinegar, and strong alcoholic beverages, especially those produced from sugar or mixed with sugared beverages.

## ADDITIONAL SUGGESTIONS

- Cooking oil should be vegetables quality only, with natural cold-pressed sesame (light or dark) and olive as preferred varieties.

- Salt should be naturally processed white sea salt.

- Traditional nonchemical shoyu or tamari soy sauce (especially for those with gluten sensitivities) and miso may be used as seasonings.

Recommended condiments include:

- Gomashio (sesame seed salt made from about 18–20 parts roasted sesame seeds to 1 part sea salt)
- Sea vegetable powder or flakes, including green nori, dulse, kelp, wakame, and others, as well as combinations and blends.
- Sesame seed wakame powder
- Umeboshi plum
- Tekka
- Roasted seeds such as sunflower or pumpkin

Pickled vegetables made without sugar or strong spice, including non-pasteurized organic sauerkraut, pickled Chinese cabbage, and others, may be eaten on a daily basis.

**IMPORTANCE OF COOKING** Proper cooking is very important for health and well being. Everyone should learn to cook either by attending classes or under the guidance of an experienced macrobiotic cook. The recipes included in macrobiotic cookbooks may also be used in planning meals.

## Way of Eating Suggestions

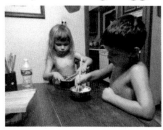

To establish health and well-being, Standard Macrobiotic Dietary practice recommends the following suggestions:

• You may eat regularly two to three times per day, as   much as is comfortable, provided the proportion of

each category of food is generally correct and in daily consumption each mouthful is thoroughly chewed

- Proper chewing is essential to digestion and it is recommended that each mouthful of food be chewed fifty times or more or until it becomes liquid in form
- Eat when you are hungry, but it is best to leave the table feeling satisfied but not full. Similarly, drink only when thirsty
- Avoid eating for three hours before sleeping, as this causes stagnation in the intestines and throughout the body
- Before and after each meal, express your gratitude verbally or silently to nature, the universe, or God who created the food and reflect on the health and happiness it is dedicated to achieving. This acknowledgment may take the form of grace, prayer, chanting, or a moment of silence. Express your thanks to parents, grandparents, and past generations who nourished us and whose dream we embody, to the vegetables or animals who gave their lives so we may live, and to the farmer, shopkeeper, and cook who contributed their energies to making the food available
- Eat regularly, two to three meals a day. When very physically active, the frequency of meals may be increased to four times a day
- Every meal should include whole grains or grain products. Grain and grain products ideally comprise about 40 to 50% of the daily intake of food
- Variety in food selection and preparation, proper combinations of foods, and proper cooking are essential
- Cooking is to be done with a peaceful mind with love, and with care
- Snacks are to be eaten in moderation. They should not replace a regular meal
- Beverages may be consumed comfortably as desired
- Refrain from eating before bedtime, preferably three hours, to allow for proper digestion
- Try to chew each mouthful very well, at least 50 times, until it becomes liquid
- Volume of food varies according to individual need

- Eat with the spirit of gratitude and appreciation for all people, society, nature, and the universe as a whole

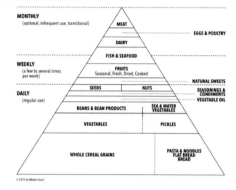

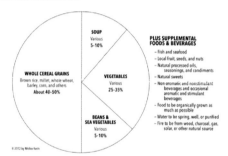

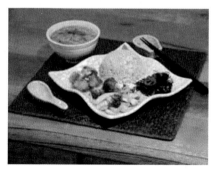

A typical macrobiotic meal consists of whole grains, miso soup, beans or bean products, vegetables from land and sea, pickles, tea, and fruit or a naturally sweetened dessert

## Kitchenware

Cooking utensils should be made from natural and durable materials as much as possible such as wood, bamboo, glass, stainless steel and cast-iron, while some materials including plastic, aluminum, copper, and non-stick coatings that may leach into food are to be avoided. A natural flame from gas, wood, charcoal, solar other natural source that gives a slow, steady source of energy is recommended, while electric ovens and microwaves create a weaker, more chaotic vibration in the food should be avoided or minimized.[7]

## Lifestyle Guidelines

Macrobiotics promotes living in harmony with nature and striving for harmony and balance in all domains of life. The three pillars of health are 1) daily diet, 2) proper exercise or physical activity, and 3) intellectual or artistic pursuits, self-reflection, or spiritual practice. Standard way of life suggestions include:

- **Live Happily and Keep Active** Live each day happily without being pre-occupied with your health. Try to keep mentally and physically active.
- **Be Grateful** View everything and everyone you meet with gratitude, particularly offering thanks before and after every meal
- **Early to Bed, Early to Rise** It is best to get up early and go to bed before midnight
- **Wear Natural Fabrics** It is best to wear cotton and other natural fiber clothing, especially for undergarments, and to use cotton bed sheets and pillows. Avoid GMO cotton and synthetic or woolen clothing directly on the skin and avoid excessive metallic accessories on the fingers, wrists, or neck. Keep such ornaments simple and graceful
- **Go Outside and Keep Home in Order** If your strength permits, go outdoors in simple clothing. Walk on the grass, beach, or soil up to one half hour each day. Keep your home in good order, from the kitchen, bathroom, bedroom, and living room, to every corner
- **Keep in Touch** Initiate and maintain an active correspondence, extending best wishes to parents, children, brothers and sisters, and friends by ordinary mail, email, texting, Skype, or phone
- **Avoid Long Bathing** Avoid taking long, hot baths or showers unless you have been consuming too much salt or animal food, as these take minerals from the body
- **Be Active** If your condition permits, exercise regularly as part of daily life, including activities like walking, scrubbing floors, cleaning windows, washing clothes, and working in the garden. You may also engage in exercise programs such as yoga, martial arts, dance, or sports

- **Minimize Electronics** Minimize the frequent use of television, computers, cell phones, and other electronics that emit artificial electromagnetic radiation
- **Oxygenate Your Home with Green Plants** Include some large green plants in your house to freshen and enrich the oxygen content of the air of your home
- **Be Kind to Animals** Treat animals, birds, insects, and all living things respectively
- **Sing a Happy Song** Sing a happy song every day

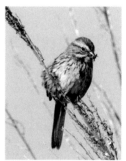

**Learn from nature.
Sing a happy song
each day**

## Progressive Development of Disease

In contrast to modern medicine that classifies disease into hundreds of categories, macrobiotic healthcare looks at sickness as a progressive pattern of seven stages:

**1. General Fatigue:** Physical tiredness, often accompanied by muscular tension and a hardening of the muscles, frequent urination and sweating, temporary constipation or diarrhea, and short periods of feeling cold or hot. Mentally we start to lose our clarity of thought, active perception and accurate responses. To recover from this stage, it usually takes a short period—from a few hours to a few days—of adequate rest, a good night's sleep, proper food and drink, and exercise.

**2. Aches and Pains:** When a feeling of general fatigue prevails, occasional pains and aches may develop. Muscular pain, headache, cramps, and various other sorts of pains and aches appear now and then. Temporary short-ness of breath, irregular heartbeat, fever and chills, and difficulty of motion also appear in this stage. Mentally, we may experience occasional depression, worry, and a general feeling of insecurity. To restore health usually takes from a few days to a few weeks, with proper dietary practice, active exercise, or necessary rest.

**3. Blood Disease:** If our dietary practice continues to be out of balance with our environment, our blood quality, including red blood cells, white blood cells, and blood plasma, becomes unsuited for maintaining harmony with our natural surroundings. The quality of our blood determines the quality of our body's cells and tissues, organs, and systems. Blood disorders create various abnormal conditions in our body from which symptoms of sickness then arise. Acidosis (a condition in which there is too much acid in the body fluids), high and low blood pressure, anemia, purpura (purple-colored spots and patches that occur on the skin caused by bleeding from small blood vessels under the skin), leukemia, scurvy, and other diseases belong to this stage, including asthma, epilepsy, and skin diseases. Mentally, this stage appears as nervousness, hypersensitivity, complaining, pessimism, timidity, and loss of general direction in life. To recover from blood disorders may take between 10 days and three to four months, depending upon the individual condition. Once again, proper dietary practices, as well as suitable exercise and rest, need to be implemented. Simple home cares to promote active circulation of the blood may also be required in some cases.

**4. Emotional Disorder:** If an improper quality of blood circulates for a prolonged period, various emotional disorders start to appear. Short temper, excitement, anger, frustration, melancholy, and a general feeling of despair are experienced frequently in daily life. A gentle approach to a problem with clear, balanced understanding is no longer possible. A general feeling of fear prevails toward new situations and surroundings, and our daily behavior and way of thinking become extremely defensive or offensive. Our physical movements become more rigid, and we gradually lose flexibility in both body and mind. It requires between one month and several months to overcome these emotional and physical disorders. Dietary change toward more balanced food is essential, along with physical and mental relaxation.

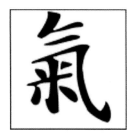

The ideogram for Ki, or life energy, is the steam rising from cooked rice. Illness is known in the East as "bad Ki" often arising from poor food choices

**5. Organ Disease** An imbalanced quality of blood circulating for a pro- longed period further produces gradual changes in the quality and function of our organs and glands. Structural change, malfunction, and degeneration start to arise. Atherosclerosis (a hardening of the arteries), diabetes, stone formation in the kidneys or gallbladder, arthritis, various types of cancer, diabetes, various types of cancer, and many other chronic diseasesfall in this category. Mentally, chronic stubbornness, prejudice, narrow-mindedness, and general rigidity with a distorted view of life become more apparent. To recover from this level of disease usually takes several months to one year or more, through continuous practice of proper diet and reorientation of the way of life, including deep self-reflection.

**6. Nervous Disorder:** From the stage of organ and gland disease, the degenerative tendency progresses toward various nervous disorders including physical paralysis, Alzheimer's disease, and mental illness including bipolar disease, schizophrenia, and paranoia. Physical and mental coordination of various functions gradually diminishes. A negative view begins to dominate daily life, and suicidal or destructive tendencies frequently manifest. It takes six months to a few years to recover completely from this stage and to regain self-assurance and trust as well as a positive view of life. The way of life has to be changed completely, including dietary practice, more harmonious relationship with the environment, and active physical exercise, together with loving care by family and friends.

**7. Self-Centeredness** An improper way of life that has been practiced for many years, finally reaches the highest level of sickness—self-centeredness or arrogance—though some of the previous stages may not have been clearly experienced. Self-centeredness is the most developed sickness and also the one that most universally affects people's lives today. Selfishness, egocentricity, vanity, self-pride, exclusivity, and self-justification are some of the common symptoms. It is the last stage of sickness and, at the same time, it is the cause of all previous stages. To overcome this attitude takes from a few years to an indefinite length of time of proper practice in a more appreciative and natural way of life. However, it can also be cured instantaneously through strong emotional or spiritual experiences, especially in the face of great difficulties and failure. The cure of self-centeredness immediately produces a spirit of humility and modesty. It restores also the spirit of appreciation through the recognition of our ignorance. When arrogance is dissolved, a new way of life in harmony with the environment automatically begins.

As Michio Kushi observed, "Every physical, mental, and spiritual sickness belongs to one of the seven levels outlined above, though symptoms at some of the steps may remain dormant and unrecognized. All sicknesses are interdependent and interconnected with one another; they are symptoms branching out from the same root—improper way of life. As long as we follow and live according to the laws of nature and the Order of the Universe, as our ancestors have done from the beginning, we shall enjoy health, happiness, and longevity, rarely suffering from any form of sickness."[8]

# The Spiral of Natural Healing

From the "macro" or largest view, macrobiotics embraces all the diverse traditions and products of human culture and tradition, including modern medicine and new nutritional and energetic techniques. The Spiral of Healing, created by Michio Kushi, illustrates the seven levels of healing:

**1. Daily Way of Eating.** At the center of the Spiral of Healing is dietary practice, namely, the macrobiotic way of eating. This approach itself is constantly evolving to take into account changing environmental and climactic conditions, social and economic factors, and personal needs. It comprises the foundation of healing.

**2. Home Remedies:** In principle, a balanced daily way of eating will help prevent sickness and harm. But if imbalance arises, special dishes, special drinks, and home remedies (most of which are based on traditional foods such as the ginger compress, ume-sho-kuzu drink, and cabbage leaf plaster) represent the next, or second circle of healing.

**3. Natural Lifestyle:** The third circle represents natural lifestyle approaches and includes simple activities and exercises that can be used to strengthen mind and body, stimulate energy flow, and promote better metabolism at various levels. Examples: do-in, or self-massage, yoga, tai chi and qi gong, walking, painting and drawing, dance, singing, playing or listening to music, prayer, meditation, mind control, and other simple, basic practices that can be performed by oneself easily, safely, and without any special cost.

**4. Natural Energy Adjustments:** The fourth level of healing involves natural energy adjustments. Examples include acupuncture (the use of needles to stimulate energy flow), moxibustion (the use of a dried herb for similar purposes), shiatsu or massage that makes use of clay or oils, aromatherapy, chiropractic, osteopathy, neurolinguistic programming, and others. Again, these external applications may be helpful depending on the case, but they generally require a second person to administer, usually an expert, and involve specialized diagnosis and evaluation, and entail an expense. Compared to the first three circles, level four represents moving beyond self-reliance to dependence on authorities, companies, and health claims that may or may not be true and beneficial.

**5. Supplements and Special Products.** The fifth circle of healing includes supplements, vitamins, minerals, herbs, and other largely nutritional products. They include both traditional substances such as Chinese herbs and modern extracts such as genistein (soy-based) tablets and homeopathic tinctures. For the most part, they originate from natural plants or animals, but the way they are processed may be calm and peaceful (like macrobiotic cooking) or highly processed (like fast foods). They may also contain other ingredients of low quality (such as gelatin, or animal-based, capsules), and they can be rather expensive and, in some cases, require an expert to prescribe or administer.

**6. Electromagnetic Treatments.** The sixth circle includes electric, radionic, digital, and other electromagnetic gadgets, devices, and machines. Again, these external applications may be helpful for any given person, but they may not be suitable for others and are often invasive, require experts, and incur significant cost.

**7. Conventional Medicine.** The seventh circle includes conventional medical procedures. The most innocuous are blood tests, EKGs, and other simple lab tests. A variety of pills, drugs, and medications carries moderate to high risks, especially SSRI's and other psychiatric drugs. Other risky procedures include surgery (which may range from mild to life-threatening, but which can damage meridian flow), radiation of different kinds (MRIs, CT scans, X-rays, mammograms), chemotherapy, and many experimental medications. Except for accidents, emergencies, and life-and-death situations, many medical procedures are unnecessary, aimed at destroying disease rather than identifying the underlying cause of imbalance. However, in any given case, they may be beneficial (especially temporarily and in small, controlled amounts or frequencies), necessary, or lifesaving.

The Spiral of Healing encourages us to develop our intuition, starting at the center and taking as much responsibility as we can for our own health and well-being. However, it prompts us to use wider, more complex methods and procedures as necessary. It is common sense to keep an open mind to all manner of healing but also to use the invasive, risky, and costly ones as a last, rather than a first, resort.

# Food as Medicine

Food has been used medicinally by all traditional cultures and civilizations. As the Hippocratic proverb puts it, "Let food by thy medicine, and thy medicine be food." Traditionally, as the below chart shows, specific tastes and foods were associated with nourishing or harming specific organs, systems, and functions of the body and consumed in whole or minimally processed form in daily meals or as home remedies.

Keep in mind that sickness or imbalance is rarely the result of taking too much of one food or not enough of another. It is the overall energetic balance that is important. The basic macrobiotic dietary approach described above will generally create optimal health and well-being and protect against illness. If specific conditions arise because of binging and taking improper food, or from lifestyle, environmental, or emotional factors, slightly increased consumption of certain foods and beverages may help tonify or improve the affected organ or function. Conversely, too much of the same item may hinder it, so moderation is the key.

For example, the top row Grains in the chart shows that maize, quinoa, and long-grain rice is especially strengthening for the heart and circulatory system, while (as the last row at the bottom suggests), beef, sugar, alcohol, and too much spice in a temperate climate weaken it. Other good foods for the heart are red lentils, kidney beans, collards, apricots, and olive oil, as well as a touch of foods with a bitter taste. Again, it is important not to eat only these foods for heart problems but just a slight amount more (2-5%) day to day. Good home remedies for the heart include Carrot-Daikon Drink that helps the body discharge excessive fat, oil, and other build up in the circulatory system, as well as Leafy Greens Drink.

# Culinary Medicine
## *Correspondences with Systems, Organs & Functions*

| | Liver, Gallbladder, Thyroid | Heart, Small Intestine, Circulatory & Nervous Systems, Brain, Pituitary & Pineal Glands | Spleen, Lymph, Pancreas, Stomach, Digestive System | Lungs, Large Intestine, Respiratory System, Microbiome | Kidney, Bladder, Reproductive System, Adrenals, Ovary, Testis |
|---|---|---|---|---|---|
| **Taste** | sour | bitter | sweet | Pungent, spicy | salty, savory, umami |
| **Grains** | barley, oats, wheat, spelt, rye, hato mugi | maize, quinoa, wild rice, long-grain and basmati rice, amaranth, sorghum, teff | millet, sweet rice | short- and medium-grain brown rice | buckwheat |
| **Grain products** | udon, couscous, bulgur, sourdough bread, fu | pancakes, crepes, tortillas, polenta, chapatis | masa | bread, crackers, muffins, pastries, mochi | soba noodles, seitan |
| **Beans** | green and French lentils, tempeh, tofu, natto | Red lentil, kidney, lima, broad, fava | chickpeas, pinto, yellow soybean | white beans | azuki, black soybean, dried tofu |
| **Vegetables** | leek, scallion, sprouts, celery, napa, bok choy | collard, lettuce, mustard greens, yellow squash, zucchini, fresh green peas | onion, cabbage, winter squash, pumpkin, parsnip, rutabaga | carrot, daikon, burdock, lotus root, broccoli, cauliflower, red radish, watercress, parsley, brussels sprouts, kale | dried daikon, dried shiitake kuzu, dried lotus, burdock |
| **Sea Veggies** | wakame | nori, dulse, agar-agar | arame, sea palm | hijiki | kombu |

| | | | | | |
|---|---|---|---|---|---|
| **Fruits** | Sour plum, sour cherry, sour apple, lemon, raspberries | watermelon, tropical fruits, blueberries, citrus fruit, strawberry | peach, apricots, sweet cherries, cantaloupe | Apple, pear, grapes, quince | blackberry, dried fruit, raisin |
| **Seeds** | flax | Poppy | Sunflower, pumpkin | light sesame | dark sesame |
| **Nuts** | peanut, hazelnut, pistachio | walnut, Brazil nut, macadamia | almond, cashew, chestnut | pine nut | water chestnut |
| **Seasonings** | vinegar, umeboshi plum, light miso, many herbs | sake, hot spices | mirin | ginger, shoyu other long-fermented food, wasabi, horseradish, smoked flavors | sea salt, tamari, dark miso |
| **Oils** | safflower, grape seed | corn, sunflower, olive | light sesame | pumpkin seed, walnut | dark sesame |
| **Condiments** | scallions with miso, wakame condiment, sauerkraut | shiso, nori and dulse flakes | nori condiment | gomashio, tekka | seaweed powders |
| **Sweeteners** | barley malt, amazake, maple syrup | honey, sugar, coconut sugar, palm sugar, molasses | fruit juice | brown rice syrup | fruit jam |
| **Beverages** | barley tea, green tea, dandelion tea, apple kukicha, lemonade, green juice, soymilk, beer | grain coffee | amazake, millet tea | bancha twig tea, brown rice tea | spring and well water, kombu tea |

| Extreme foods and sub-stances (to be avoided or mini-mized) | lamb, goat, milk, soft cheese, ice cream, yogurt, shellfish, palm oil, coconut oil, canola oil | beef, active ocean fish, trop-ical fruits and vegetables, sugar, chocolate, cof-fee, herbs, spic-es, dry wine, alcohol, drugs | chicken, but-ter, smaller ocean fish, sweet wine | eggs, salty cheese, to-bacco, very compact ocean fish such as tuna, salmon, sar-dine | table salt, pork, trout, perch, flounder, and other fresh-water fish |
|---|---|---|---|---|---|

# Scientific and Medical Studies

## The World's First Nutritional Experiment

The opening story in the Book of Daniel in the Bible is the world's oldest nutrition experiment.

### ☤ The Book of Daniel

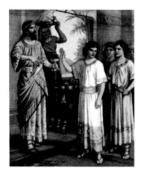

**Young Daniel requests a simple, grain-based diet at the palace of the King of Babylon**

During the Babylonian Captivity, King Nebu-chadnezzar commanded several of the most gifted young men of Israel to be brought to court to enter the royal service. The king in-structed Malasar, the master of his household, to feed Daniel and his three companions the best meat and wine from the royal table. The Israelites, however, refused the rich food and instead asked for the simple meals they were accustomed to. The steward rejected their request, fearing that he would lose his head if the king saw Daniel and his friends undernour-ished in comparison to the young Babylonians their age also in training for royal service. Dan-iel replied: "Try, I beseech thee, thy servants for ten days, and let pulse [whole grains, len-tils, seeds] be given us to eat, and water to drink. And look upon our fac-es, and the faces of the children that eat of the king's meat: and as thou shalt see, deal with thy servants. And when he had heard these words, he tried them for ten days. And after ten days their faces appeared fairer and fatter than all the children that ate of the king's meat. So Malasar took their portions, and the wine that they should drink: and he gave them pulse. And to these children God gave knowledge and understanding in every book, and wisdom: but to Daniel the understanding also of all visions and dreams."[9]

As the world's first nutrition experiment, the episode involves two groups (an intervention group of young Jews and a control group of young Babylonians), dietary variables (a plant vs. animal-based diet), a set duration (10 days), observable outcomes (change in countenance, disposition, and physique), and an impartial investigator (steward of the palace of the king of Babylon). As a result of his macrobiotic diet and divine favor, Daniel became the principal adviser to the King, a great prophet, and leader who helped deliver his people from captivity.

## Macrobiotic & Whole Foods Nutrition

Over the years, scientific and medical studies have generally found that the macrobiotic way of eating meets current nutritional guidelines. These studies include:

### ♼ Landmark Report Links Diet with Degenerative Disease

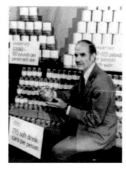

Senator George McGovern shows the harmful effects of sugar and soft drinks on public health

Summarizing its conclusions on the nation's way of eating, health, and future direction, the historic Senate report, *Dietary Goals for the United States* (also known as the McGovern Report after its chairman, former Democratic presidential candidate George McGovern) launched the modern nutritional revolution in 1977: "During this century, the composition of the average diet in the United States has changed radically. Complex carbohydrates— fruit, vegetables, and grain products—which were the mainstay of the diet, now play a minority role. At the same time, fat and sugar consumption have risen to the point where these two dietary elements alone now comprise at least 60 percent of total calorie intake, up from 50 percent in the early 1900s. In the view of doctors and nutritionists consulted by the Select Committee, these and other changes in the diet amount to a wave of malnutrition—of both over- and underconsumption—that may be as profoundly damaging to the Nation's health as the widespread contagious diseases of the early part of this century. The overconsumption of fat, generally, and saturated fat in particular, as well as cholesterol, sugar, salt, and alcohol have been related to six of the leading causes of death: Heart disease, cancer, cerebrovascular diseases, diabetes, arteriosclerosis, and cirrhosis of the liver."

Macrobiotic educators Michio and Aveline Kushi; the East West Foundation under the leadership of Edward Esko and Stephen Uprichard; and *East West Journal* under Sherman Goldman, Alex Jack, and Tom Monte wrote about the relationship of diet and degenerative disease and prepared materials or met with key experts and witnesses in the hearings.[10]

## Macrobiotic Practice Meets Nutritional Guidelines

Researchers at the University of Rhode Island studied 76 macrobiotic people and reported in the *Journal of the American Dietetic Association* in 1980 they met currently acceptable medical and nutritional guidelines, including mean values for hemoglobin, hematocrit, serum iron, and transferrin saturation, serum ascorbic acid, vitamin A, beta-carotene, riboflavin, vitamin B-12, and folate.[11]

## Macrobiotic Diet Meets or Exceeds British RDAs

At the University of London, researchers measured the dietary intakes of 10 people practicing macrobiotics and they were found to be adequate in all major nutrients of the United Kingdom Recommended Daily amounts. All of the other nutrients either met the RDA's or, in the case of vitamins A and C, thiamine, calcium, and iron, "far exceeded the recommendations." "The macrobiotic diet as eaten by the participants of this study was found to conform with many of the recommendations put forward by recent [medical and scientific] reports on eating for health," according to the chief researcher's report in 1985.[12]

## The China Study

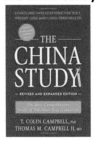

The world's most comprehensive nutrition study supports a macrobiotic way of eating. A Chinese research project, hailed as the "Grand Prix of Epidemiology," challenged modern dietary assumptions. Sponsored by the U.S. National Cancer Institute and the Chinese Institute of Nutrition and Food Hygiene, the decade-long study in the 1990s correlated average food and nutrient intakes with disease mortality rates in 65 rural Chinese counties. The typical Chinese diet included a high proportion of cereal grains and vegetables and a low content of animal food. Less than 1 percent of deaths were caused by coronary heart disease, cancer, and other chronic diseases common in the West.

Study director Dr. T. Colin Campbell, a professor of nutrition at Cornell University and member of the expert committee that developed the U.S. Food Guide Pyramid, concluded:

- **Reduce Fat** Fat consumption should ideally be reduced to 10 to 15 percent of calories to prevent degenerative disease, not 30 percent as usually recommended
- **Eat More Plant-Based Foods** The lowest risk for cancer is generated by the consumption of a variety of fresh plant products
- **Reduce Animal Protein** Eating animal protein is a main cause of chronic disease. Compared to the Chinese who derive 11 percent of their protein from animal sources, Americans obtain 70 percent from animal food
- **Natural Menstruation** A rich diet that promotes early menstruation may increase a woman's risk of cancer of the breast and reproductive organs. In the West, girls typically begin to menstruate at 11, in China at 17
- **Strengthen Bones by Avoiding Dairy** Dairy food is not needed to prevent osteoporosis, the thinning of the bones that is common
- among older women, and indeed may be a cause for bone loss
- **Eat Leafy Greens for Iron** Meat consumption is not needed to prevent iron-deficiency anemia. The average Chinese consumes twice the iron Americans do, primarily from plant sources, and show no signs of anemia

Dr. Campbell, who grew up on a dairy farm, because a vegan as a result of his studies and frequently lectures at macrobiotic conferences. The healthy traditional Chinese diet, he explains, is essentially macrobiotic.[13]

### ⚕ Higher in Iron and Other Nutrients Than Standard Diet
Researchers at the University of Memphis and University of South Carolina evaluated the dietary pattern at the Kushi Institute's Way to Health program and concluded in a 2015 article in *Nutrition and Cancer* that it had a lower percentage of potentially harmful fats, higher total dietary fiber, and higher amounts of most micronutrients, including beta-carotene, B vitamins, and iron, than the standard American diet. "Findings from this analysis of a macrobiotic diet plan indicate the potential for disease prevention and suggest the need for studies of real-world consumption as well as designing, implementing, and testing interventions based on the macrobiotic approach," the scientists concluded.[14]

### ⚕ Rich in Nutrient-Dense Foods
In an article on the popular website WebMD.com, Dr. Michael Smith observed in 2016: "If you're looking for a healthy eating plan, the macrobiotic diet is a good choice. It's rich in nutrient-packed foods that are also low in calories. While there's no absolute proof, medical research suggests diets that are mostly vegetables, fruits, and whole grains may low-

er the risk of several diseases, including heart disease and cancer. Either way, you'll reap plenty of health benefits with this diet."[15]

## Heart Disease

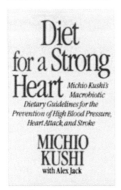

In the early 1970s, Frank Sachs, a student at Harvard Medical School, was impressed with Michio Kushi's lectures and arranged with his professors at Channing Laboratory to begin the first medical studies on macrobiotics. They focused on blood pressure, cholesterol levels, and other basic blood values. Several hundred members of the macrobiotic community volunteered for what turned out to be a series of studies that were published in the *New England Journal of Medicine, Atheroclerosis*, and other major journals. The studies convincingly linked diet and heart disease, which until then had been largely neglected, and led to the first national dietary guidelines on the number one cause of death in modern society. The macrobiotic approach, including these studies, was featured in Michio Kushi's *Diet for a Strong Heart*.

### ⚕ Boston Macrobiotics at Zero Risk for Heart Disease

In a study of 210 men and women eating a macrobiotic diet, Harvard Medical School researchers found that the men had mean systolic blood pressures of 109.7 mm Hg and diastolic pressures of 60.9. The women had 100.9 and 58.2 respectively. Both of these measurements fell well within the normal blood pressure category and approached the systolic level of 100 under which Framingham Heart Study researchers theorized there would develop virtually no coronary heart disease.[16]

### ⚕ Average Macrobiotic Cholesterol 126

Harvard Medical School researchers reported that Boston-area macrobiotic people had significantly lower cholesterol and triglyceride levels and lower blood pressure than a control group from the Framingham Heart Study eating the standard American diet of meat, sugar, dairy foods, and highly processed, chemicalized foods. The average serum cholesterol in the macrobiotic group was 126 milligrams per deciliter versus 184 for controls. "The low plasma lipid levels in the vegetarians," the researchers concluded in the *New England Journal of Medicine*, "resemble those reported for populations in non-industrialized societies" where heart disease, cancer, and other degenerative illnesses are uncommon.[17]

### ☥ Surgeon General Cites Macrobiotic Diet for Heart Health

In his annual report in 1979, the U.S. Surgeon General reported for the first time that existing coronary heart disease could be relieved by dietary measures. "Direct evidence from animal studies supports the linkage of atherosclerosis with high levels of fats (particularly saturated) and cholesterol in the diet . . . [and] that Americans who habitually eat less fat rich foods ([macrobiotic] vegetarians and Seventh Day Adventists, for example) have less heart disease than other Americans; and that atherosclerotic plaques in certain arteries may be reversed by cholesterol-lowering diets."[18]

### ☥ Pioneer Study Links Animal Food and High Blood Pressure

In one of the first studies to show the direct effects of animal food on raising blood pressure, a study of 21 macrobiotic persons by Harvard Medical School researchers in 1981 found that the addition of 250 grams of beef per day for four weeks to their regular diet of whole grains and vegetables raised serum cholesterol levels 19 percent. Systolic blood pressure also rose significantly. After returning to a low-fat diet, cholesterol and blood pressure values returned to previous levels, the researchers reported in the *Journal of the American Medical Association*).[19]

### ☥ Macrobiotic Practitioners Healthier Than Marathon Runners

William Castelli, M.D., director of the Framingham Heart Study, the nation's oldest and largest cardiovascular research project, and a participant in research on macrobiotic people at Harvard Medical School, noted that macrobiotic people have healthier hearts and circulatory systems than conditioned athletes: "What a person eats every day is a very important aspect of how his or her health will be in every day as well as later life. Supporting this view is the fact that macrobiotic people studied had a ratio [of total cholesterol to HDL cholesterol of] 2.5 and Boston marathon runners were at 3.4, ratios at which rarely, if ever, is coronary heart disease seen. Studies and observations such as these are a clear indicator that people need to take a critical look at their diet with the intention of making changes now."[20]

### ☥ Macrobiotics Aids Angina Patients in New York Hospital

Physicians at Columbia Presbyterian Hospital in New York City reported that patients with angina pectoris, showed improved blood pressure values and lowered coronary risk factors after ten weeks on a macrobiotic diet and treatment with biofeedback. Dr. Kenneth Greenspan of the hospital's Laboratory and Center for Stress Related Disorders, reported that cholesterol dropped from an average 300 to 220, levels of blood pressure also dropped, patients could walk about 20 percent farther in stress tests, and three patients with severe angina showed no symptoms at the end of the study.[21]

### ⚕ Major Mediterranean-Macrobiotic Diet Study on Metabolic Syndrome

Age-related non-communicable chronic diseases are the leading cause of mortality. Italian researchers designed a phase III randomized controlled trial to evaluate the effect of a comprehensive lifestyle intervention, including moderate physical activity and a Mediterranean-macrobiotic diet) and the effect of treatment with metformin in the prevention of chronic diseases in healthy people with metabolic syndrome, a clustering of risk factors of metabolic origin such as abdominal obesity, high blood pressure, and abnormal blood values. The double-blind 5-year study began in 2018 with two thousand volunteers randomized into 4 equal groups of five hundred each.[22]

### ⚕ Macrobiotics Aids Angina Patients in New York Hospital

In a study of forty subjects, aged 40-69, with high normal blood pressure or stage 1 hypertension, a random case control study found that miso soup intake for 8 weeks significantly reduced nighttime blood pressure without affecting pulse rate. The control group, taking soy food, did not affect blood pressure. "This is the first report showing that miso reduces nighttime blood pressure in humans," the Japanese researchers reported. "Miso may do so by shrinking the fluid spaces in the body and/or deactivating the adrenergic nervous system."[23]

### ⚕ Miso Soup Reduces Nighttime Blood Pressure

In a study of forty subects, aged 40-69, with high normal blood pressure or stage 1 hypertension, a random case control study found that miso soup intake for 8 weeks significantly reduced nighttime blood pressure without affecting pulse rate. The control group, taking soy food, did not affect blood pressure. "This is the first report showing that miso reduces nighttime blood pressure in humans," the Japanese researchers reported. "Miso may do so by shrinking the fluid spaces in the body and/or deactivating the adrenergic nervous system."[24]

## Cancer

During the 20th century, the incidence of cancer in modern society soared, rising from 2% of the population in 1900 to 25% in the 1950s and 1960s. There was no effective treatment or cure, and many people felt it marked a death sentence. In Boston, Michio Kushi began to give personal dietary and way of life consultations, and many cancer patients came to him for advice. The first person to experience complete remission following a macrobiotic way of eating was Professor Jean

Kohler, a university instructor in music at Ball State College in Indiana, who had pancreatic cancer, a nearly always fatal illness. Following his successful recovery in the late 1970s, the Kushis and their associates began to focus on cancer, especially now that the medical studies at Harvard and the Framingham Heart Study had shown that a balanced, whole foods diet could bring down high blood pressure, lower cholesterol, and reduce the risk of heart disease. [25]

The *East West Journal*, the macrobiotic monthly magazine, focused on cancer and diet, publishing macrobiotic case histories, and investigating the ties of the medical profession to the food industry. Journalist Peter Barry Chowka wrote several influential investigative articles on the American Cancer Society and National Cancer Institute and their neglect of dietary and lifestyle factors in the etiology of the disease. The East West Foundation, under the Kushis's auspices, sponsored the first Conference on Cancer and Diet, at Pine Manor College in Brookline, MA in 1978. The gathering brought together physicians, researchers, and many patients who had recovered using a macrobiotic approach. St. Martin's Press brought out Kushi's major book, *The Cancer-Prevention Diet*, co-authored by Alex Jack, editor-in-chief of *East West Journal,* in 1983. The book was translated into more than a dozen languages and included chapters on 20 major types of cancer, including a description of the food patterns underling their cause, dietary guidelines for recovery, home remedies, and lifestyle suggestions.

Over the years, hundreds—possibly thousands—of people, recovered from cancer with the help of macrobiotics. At the Kushi Institute in Becket, Massachusetts, the main residential center for macrobiotic education, the one-week Way to Health Program introduced individuals and families, many with cancer or other chronic diseases, to the principles and practices of macrobiotic, including daily cooking classes, menu planning, and proper use of home remedies. Many people who met with Michio Kushi or other counselors, or who attended programs at the K.I. (or affiliated campuses around the world) went on to lead healthy, fulfilling lives and chronicled their healing stories in their own books or articles. These included:

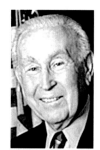

- **Businessman Heals Pancreatic Cancer** Norman Arnold, a businessman from South Carolina, who recovered from pancreatic cancer. He went on to live cancer-free for another 35 years and establish the Cancer Center at the University of South Carolina that employed several macrobiotic-oriented researchers.[26]
- **Journalist Heals Metastatic Ovarian and Lymph Cancer** Milenka Dobic, a journalist from Yugoslavia with ovarian and lymph cancer. She went on to become a leading macrobiotic teacher and counselor and described her recovery in *My Beautiful Life*.[27]

**Norman Arnold recovered from pancreatic cancer**

- **Hollywood Star Recovers from Prostate Cancer** Dirk Benedict, the actor and star of *The A-Team* and *Battlestar Galactica*, who recovered from prostate cancer.[28]
- **Mother Overcomes Inoperable Uterine Tumor** Elaine Nussbaum, a mother from New Jersey with an inoperable uterine tumor, who went on to become a leading macrobiotic teacher and cook.[29]
- **United Nations Official Recovers from Stomach Cancer** Katsuhide Kitatani, deputy Secretary-General of the United Nations, who had stomach cancer. He went on to found the U.N. Macrobiotic Society and 2050, a nonprofit development organization in Southeast Asia.[30]
- **Brain Tumor Overcome** Mona Sanders, a young woman from Columbus, Mississippi, had a brain tumor. After recovering, she served as an assistant to Michio Kushi and moved to India, where she taught diet and health for the next 25 years.[31]
- **Physician and Hospital President Heals Prostate Cancer** Anthony Sattilaro, M.D., president of Methodist Hospital in Philadelphia, who had metastatic prostate cancer that spread to the bones, testicles, and other internal organs. Within a few weeks of starting a macrobiotic diet, the back pain he suffered for years eased, and after several months his tumors went away. One-year and four-year follow up scans at his own hospital confirmed that the cancer had completely disappeared. Dr. Sattilaro was profiled in *East West Journal, Saturday Evening Post* and *Life* magazines and went on to write a bestselling book with Tom Monte *Recalled By Life.*[32]

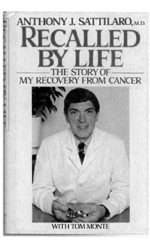

- **Leukemia Survivor Turned Celebrity Chef** Christina Pirello, a young woman with leukemia, married her macrobiotic counselor, Bob Pirello, and went on to become a macrobiotic teacher, chef, and Emmy-award winning star of the longtime PBS-TV show *Christina Cooks!*[33]
- **Nurse Overcomes Metastatic Lung Cancer** Janet E. Vitt, R.N., a nurse in Cleveland, had stage 4 lung cancer that had spread to her liver, pancreas, abdomen, and lymph system. After exhausting her medical options, she went to a mac-

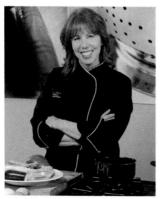

After healing herself of leukemia, Christina Pirello became host of PBS's *Christina Cooks*

robiotic counselor and after 10 months the tumors were all gone. Jane went on to become a macrobiotic cook, teacher, and counselor, guiding many people to greater health and well-being.[34]

- **Nurse Reverses Malignant Melanoma** Virginia Brown, R.N., a nurse in Vermont, recovered from malignant melanoma. Her story appeared in *Macrobiotic Miracle*.[35]
- **Physician Documents Husband's Recovery from Colon Cancer** Vivian Newbold, M.D., a Philadelphia physician chronicled the recovery of her husband who had colon cancer.[36]
- **Businessman Heals Prostate Cancer** Ken Walles, a Long Island businessman, healed himself of prostate cancer with the help of macrobiotics.[37]

Personal accounts are among the most powerful and convincing testimony on the benefits of macrobiotics. However, for the medical community, these claims needed to be evaluated scientifically. Over the years, there have been studies of the macrobiotic approach to cancer by the NIH, CDC, and other medical organizations and research centers:

### NIH Best Case Series of 77 Macrobiotic Cancer Recoveries
The National Institute of Health's (NIH) Macrobiotic Best Case Series undertaken by researchers at the University of Minnesota in the 1990s, documented the medical histories of 77 individuals who recovered from cancer with the help of macrobiotics. These included cancers of the prostate (20 cases), breast (12 cases), malignant melanoma (8), lymphoma (8), leukemia (6), astrocytoma (5), colorectal (4), endometrium (3), ovary (3), pancreas (3), kidney (2), liver (1), small cell lung (1), multiple myeloma (1), nose plasmacytoma (1), parotic gland (1), sarcoma (1), and small intestine (1).[38]

### NCI Approves Clinical Study on Macrobiotics and Cancer
The Cancer Advisory Panel on Complementary and Alternative Medicine (CAPCAM), an expert committee of oncologists from the National Institute of Cancer (NCI), in 2003 reviewed the cases of six persons who had been diagnosed with IVth stage metastasized cancer and were part of the NIH Best Cases Series. The review included viewing patient slides and records, hearing expert testimony from a radiologist and pathologist, and listening to an explanation on macrobiotic theory and practice by Michio Kushi. In addition, three of the six persons whose cases were being reviewed gave personal testimony and answered questions from the panelists. At the end of a day-long, rigorous review, the panel of 15 physicians and scientists voted unanimously to recommend

to the NCI that governmental funding should be provided for a prospective and full clinical study on macrobiotics and cancer.[39]

### ☤ CDC Reviews 51 Macrobiotic Healing Cases
In a study sponsored by the Centers for Disease Control and Disease Prevention (CDC), the public health arm of the United States, cancer researchers at the School of Public Health, University of South Carolina, investigated the macrobiotic way of life from 2000-2002. In a report "Macrobiotics in the United States: An Assessment of Services and Activities," Sheldon and Ginat Rice interviewed 124 practitioners in 44 locales. Fifty-one people recounted personal healing stories in which macrobiotic practice reversed a serious health condition. Of these, twenty-one were instances of cancer and four more were pre-cancerous cysts. The researchers posted a selection of recovery stories from cancer and other chronic diseases on the Internet along with a list of macrobiotic resources, including educational centers, teachers and counselors, and books and other study materials for the use of the general public.[40]

### ☤ M.D. Anderson Cancer Center Reviews Macrobiotics
Cancer researchers at M.D. Anderson Cancer Center at the University of Texas in Houston posted a historical overview of macrobiotics as a therapy for cancer patients and the general public on their web site in early 2003. "The macrobiotic diet is part of a way of life that attempts to achieve balance by applying the oriental principles of yin and yang to the selection of foods. According to one study, 63% of cancer patients who received some form of dietary therapy received or were exposed to the macrobiotic diet."[41]

## Breast Cancer
Breast cancer is the most common form of cancer in American women, and about 1 in 8 will contract this disease. Many women have recovered following a macrobiotic approach, and medical studies found that the diet leads to improved processing of estrogen and other hormones and improved microflora in the gut:

### ☤ Macrobiotic Women Less Likely to Develop Breast Cancer
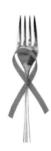
Macrobiotic and vegetarian women are less likely to develop breast cancer, researchers at New England Medical Center in Boston reported in 1981. The scientists found that macrobiotic and vegetarian women process estrogen differently from other women and eliminate it more quickly from their body. "The difference in estrogen metabolism may ex-

plain the lower incidence of breast cancer in vegetarian [macrobiotic] women," the study published in *Cancer Research* concluded.[42]

### ⚕ Kombu Protects Against Breast Cancer

Jane Teas, Ph.D., a researcher at Harvard University, and her colleagues found that kombu, a thick green seaweed that is a part of the regular macrobiotic way of eating, protected against breast cancer in laboratory studies.[43] In another study, a Japanese researcher reported that rats fed sea vegetables had about half the induced breast cancer rate than controls.[44]

### ⚕ Macrobiotic Diet Reduces Hormonal Levels in Italian Women

In a random case con-trol study involving 104 middle-aged women at high risk for breast can-cer, researchers at the National Tumor Insti-tute in Milan, Italy, re-ported that a macrobi-otic diet could substan-tially reduce hormonal levels associated with higher risk for this ma-lignancy. The interven-tion group lost more weight, 4.06 kg com-

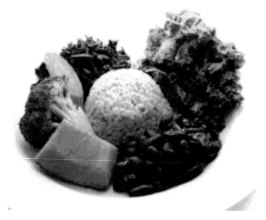

Breast cancer risk fell on a macrobiotic diet.

pared to 0.54 kg, and underwent statistically significant improvements in the five major hormonal and metabolic values associated with breast cancer risk: sex hormone-binding globulin, testosterone, estradiol, fast-ing insulin, and fasting glycemia. Serum sex hormone-binding globulin levels increased 25.2%, while testosterone and estradiol decreased 19.5% and 18%."We observed significant and favorable changes in hor-monal indicators of breast cancer risk in a group of postmenopausal women living in northern Italy," the researchers concluded. "These re-sults suggest that the multifactorial dietary intervention applied in this study may prevent breast cancer if continued in the long term." "Com-pared with the usual Western microflora, the gut of macrobiotic or vege-tarian subjects may be richer in lactobacilli and bifidobacteria," the sci-entists noted in an article in *Cancer Epidemiology, Biomarkers, & Preven-tion*. The study led to a series of further studies on the effectiveness of the macrobiotic approach to this illness.[45]

## ☤ Diet Lowers Risk of BRCA Breast Cancer

A plant-based diet lowers the risk of breast cancer for women who test positive for BRCA. In a review of the medical literature, Alex Jack found that a plant-based diet resulted in lower IGF-1 levels (reducing risk up to 7 times or 85%) among women testing positive for the BRCA gene mutation.[46] Higher consumption of fruits and vegetables reduced risk between 72 and 82%.[47] Lower weight brought the risk down between 80 and 90%. Breastfeeding reduced risk by 45% (BRCA1 type only).[48] He concluded that the well-publicized case of Angelina Jolie who had a double mastectomy was especially tragic because she had already altered her diet and breastfed her children, bringing her risk down to normal. Her doctors told her without surgery she had an 87% higher risk of breast or ovarian cancer. Neither Jolie nor her doctors appear to have known of these studies.

About 1-2% of women of Scandinavian, Icelandic, Dutch, and Ashkenazi Jewish heritage carry the BRCA mutation. Jack hypothesized that the BRCA, a normal DNA repair gene, mutated several centuries ago when dairy food consumption in these regions increased as society became more affluent. As macrobiotics has long contended, dairy food is a main cause of breast cancer. The Nurses' Health Study II found premenopausal women who ate a lot of high-fat dairy products (like whole milk or butter) had an increased risk of breast cancer.[49] Researchers in California reported breast cancer patients who eat a singe portion of cheese, yogurt, or ice cream daily could be 50% more likely to die. Scientists from the Kaiser Permanente research center in California looked at the records of 1,500 women diagnosed with breast cancer between 1997 and 2000 and concluded that the hormone estrogen found in milk and other dairy products encourages tumor growth.[50]

The BRCA genes are genes that repair chromosomal damage in DNA double-strand breaks. The more milk, cheese, and dairy consumed, the more genetic abnormalities arise, Jack theorized, causing the BRCA repair genes to work harder to repair them. Eventually they become impeded or worn out, mutated, and become ineffective. Scandinavians and the Dutch are well-known consumers of dairy food. In the case of those of Ashkenazi Jewish descent, bagels and cream cheese, cheese blintzes, cheesecake, and cottage cheese, originated in Central and Eastern Europe and were Ashkenazi staples.

From an epigenetic perspective, it appears excessive milk, cheese, and other dairy intake caused hypermethylation or abnormal histone changes at the gene level that were passed along from mother to daughter. Today, BRCA mutations are found in tiny percentages in people of virtually all backgrounds and nationalities, including African-Americans, Native Americans, Pakistanis, and Japanese. By observing the modern food pattern, high in dairy and other cancer-promoting foods such as sugar, women around the world are developing similar epigenetic changes for the worse.[51]

## Colon Cancer

Along with lung cancer, colon cancer is the most deadly malignancy for both men and women. In addition to a balanced, plant-based diet, special remedies may be effective to help relieve this condition.

### ⚕ Daikon a Potent Food for Colon Cancer

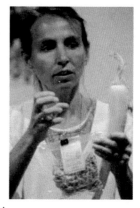

Daikon, the large white radish used in traditional Far Eastern cooking, has chemopreventive properties. In a study published in the *Journal of Agriculture and Food Chemistry*, researchers reported that an extract of daikon inhibited three lines of human colon cancer cells. Daikon is used regularly in macrobiotic cooking. For many years, educator Michio Kushi has recommended a special Daikon Carrot Drink to help relieve colon cancer and other malignancies. Native to the East, daikon is now grown in North America, Europe, and throughout the world.[52]

**Bettina Zumdick shows the healing properties of daikon radish**

## Endometrial Cancer

Soy foods are high in isoflavones, naturally occurring compounds that protect from illness. Many medical studies have shown that a diet high in traditionally processed soy (as opposed to soy supplements, analogues, and GMO soy) reduce the risk for female disorders, including endometrial conditions, breast cancer, and reproductive disorders.

### ⚕ Tofu and Legumes May Reduce Endometrial Cancer Risk

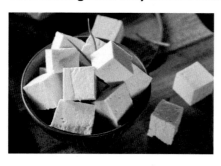

**Tofu is a high-protein soy product that is good for both daily health and for healing**

Phytochemicals in tofu, legumes, and other soy and legume products reduce the risk of endometrial cancer. University of Hawaii Cancer Center researchers observed 489 non-hysterectomized postmenopausal women with this malignancy over 13.6 years. Reduce endometrial cancer risk was associated with total isoflavone intake, and increasing intake of tofu or soy did not increase risk.[53] The macrobiotic way has also been helpful for women suffering from endometriosis.

## Lung Cancer

Miso and other traditionally made soy foods may help prevent or relieve lung cancer.

### ☤ Miso Soup and Other Soy Foods Inhibit Lung Cancer

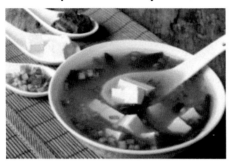
**Miso inhibits tumor development**

In Japan, soy is consumed in a wide variety of forms, such as miso soup and soy sauce. In a study to investigate the effect of genistein, an isoflavone found in soy, on osteosarcoma cells, Japanese researchers reported in 2012 that miso and other soy foods high in genistein inhibited cell proliferation, especially in the lungs. It decreased invasive and motile potential by inducing cell differentiation. "Genistein may be useful as an anti-metastatic drug for osteosarcoma," the researchers concluded.[54]

## Pancreatic Cancer

Pancreatic cancer has the poorest prognosis of all major types of cancer. As the cases of Jean Kohler, Norman Arnold, and others noted above show, it has lent itself to macrobiotic recoveries. The following medical study was inspired by these successes:

### ☤ Pancreatic Patients Live Nearly 3 Times Longer

Researchers at Tulane University reported that the 1-year survival rate among patients with pancreatic cancer was significantly higher among those who adopted a macrobiotic diet than among those who did not (17 months versus 6 months). The one-year survival rate was 54.2 percent in the macrobiotic patients versus 10.0 percent in the controls. "This exploratory analysis suggests that a strict macrobiotic diet is more likely to be effective in the long-term management of cancer than are diets that provide a variety of other foods," the scientists concluded in the *American Journal of Clinical Nutrition*.[55]

## Prostate Cancer

Prostate cancer is the most prevalent cancer in American men. In addition to several well publicized accounts of personal recoveries, the macrobiotic approach has been studied by several medical researchers:

### ⚕ Prostate Patients Live Nearly Twice as Long

Tulane University researchers found that patients with metastatic prostate cancer who followed a macrobiotic diet lived longer (177 months compared to 91 months) and enjoyed an improved quality of life than controls. The researchers concluded that the macrobiotic approach could be an effective adjunctive treatment to conventional treatment or in primary management of cancers with a nutritional association. "This exploratory analysis suggests that a strict macrobiotic diet is more likely to be effective in the long-term management of cancer than are diets that provide a variety of other foods," the study published in the *American Journal of Nutrition* concluded.[56]

### ⚕ PSA Levels Drop Significantly on a Macrobiotic Diet

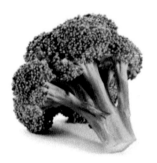

**Green vegetables help protect against prostate cancer**

At Moores Cancer Center, University of California, San Diego, researchers undertook two intervention studies of patients with recurrent prostate cancer. In a 6-month pilot clinical trial to investigate whether adoption of a modified macrobiotic diet high in whole grains, fresh vegetables, and other plant foods, reinforced by stress management training, could attenuate the rate of further rise of PSA [prostate-specific antigen, a risk factor], 14 patients with recurrent prostate cancer experienced a significant decrease in the rate of PSA rise. Four of 10 evaluable patients experienced an absolute reduction in their PSA levels, nine of ten had a reduction in their rates of PSA rise and improvement of their PSA doubling times. Mean PSA doubling time increased from 11.9 months to 112.3 months. "These results provide preliminary evidence that adoption of a plant-based [macrobiotic] diet, in combination with stress reduction, may attenuate disease progression and have therapeutic potential for clinical management of recurrent prostate cancer," the researchers reported in *Integrative Cancer Therapies* in 2006.[57]

## Stomach Cancer

Stomach tumors are linked to eating salted meats, white rice, and other foods in the modern Asian diet where this cancer is widespread.

### ⚕ Miso Protects Against Stomach Cancer and Heart Disease

Japan's National Cancer Center reported that people who eat miso soup daily are 33 percent less likely to contract stomach cancer and have 19 percent less cancer at other sites than those who never eat miso soup. The thirteen-year study, involving about 265,000 men and women over forty, also found that those who never ate miso soup had a 43 percent higher death rate from coronary heart disease than those who consumed miso soup daily. Those who abstained from miso also had 29 percent more fatal strokes, 3.5 times more deaths resulting from high blood pressure, and higher mortality from all other causes.[58]

### ⚕ Shiitake Have Strong Anti-Tumor Effect

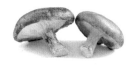

Shiitake help discharge fat and oil deposits in the body and prevent tumors

Japanese scientists at the National Cancer Center Research Institute reported that shiitake mushrooms had a strong anti-tumor effect. In experiments with mice, polysaccharide preparations from various natural sources, including the shiitake mushroom commonly available in Tokyo markets, markedly inhibited the growth of induced sarcomas resulting in "almost complete regression of tumors . . with no sign of toxicity."[59]

## General Medical Opinion

As a result of the above studies on the macrobiotic approach to cancer, major medical organizations have generally supported its potential to help prevent and, in some cases, relieve cancer:

### ⚕ American Cancer Society Lists Benefits of Macrobiotics

In a statement on alternative therapies in 1996, the American Cancer Society observed, "Today's most popular anticancer diet is probably macrobiotics." While no diet has yet been shown to be able to reverse existing tumors, the ACS went on: "Like other fat-reducing diets, macrobiotics may help prevent some cancers. It may reduce the risk of developing cancers that appear related to higher fat intake, such as colon cancer and possibly some breast cancers. The macrobiotic diet, like other fat-free diets, can lower blood pressure and perhaps reduce the chance of heart disease. Taking part in a macrobiotics program may provide some sense of balance with nature and harmony with the total universe and as such promote a sense of calmness and reduced stress." [60]

### ⚕ ACS Says Macrobiotics Assists Conventional Treatment

In advice to cancer survivors, the American Cancer Society further declared in 2003 that the macrobiotic way of eating could be beneficial. "The macrobiotic diet and lifestyle is not primarily aimed at cancer survivors, yet many persons first encounter this diet in the context of cancer. This diet is based on whole grains, vegetables, sea vegetables, beans, fermented soy products, fruit, nuts, seeds, soups, small amounts of fish, and teas. Individualized diets are based on whether a cancer is classified yin or yang. Macrobiotic diets may be used as an adjuvant to conventional treatment to ensure nutritional variety and adequacy." [61]

### ⚕ ACS Recommends a Plant-Based Diet

The American Cancer Society's *Guidelines on Nutrition and Physical Activity for Cancer-Prevention* stated that one-third of malignancies were due to diet and physical activity habits. Among its key recommendations were "Consume a healthy diet, with an emphasis on plant foods," "Choose whole grains instead of refined grain products," "Limit consumption of processed meat and red meat." [62]

### ⚕ Macrobiotic Diet Improves Drug Metabolism

In a review of complementary and alternative therapies for cancer in *American Family Physician*, a researcher reported that a macrobiotic diet may positively alter drug metabolism and that in well-nourished patients who do not have breast or endometrial cancer, "a macrobiotic diet can be accepted by the physician as an adjunct of conventional treatment." [63]

### ⚕ Oncologists Encourage Aspects of Macrobiotic Diet

In a study of the pros and cons of dietary strategies popular among cancer patients, researchers reported in *Oncology* that the macrobiotic diet met the majority of the guidelines of the American Cancer Society and the American Institute for Cancer Research. "Clinicians should consider strategies to encourage evidence-based dietary changes that encourage positive features of popular cancer diets, while minimizing negative aspects," the scientists concluded. [64]

As these studies indicate, macrobiotics opened the way for research on the dietary approach to cancer. Michio Kushi met with Dr. Mark Hegsted, a nutritionalist from Harvard, and others who influenced *Dietary Goals for the U.S.*, the historic 1977 Senate report linking the modern way of eating with heart disease, cancer, and other leading causes of death and led to the first national and international dietary guidelines for cancer. In the years that followed, macrobiotics became the most popular dietary treatment for those with this disease. Every year, these recommendations move closer to the macrobiotic approach. For example, the American Cancer Society dietary guidelines for cancer emphasizing a plant-based approach noted above were composed in 2012 by a committee chaired by Lawrence H. Kushi, ScD, an epidemiologist and breast cancer researcher, son of Michio and Aveline Kushi, and lifelong practitioner of macrobiotics.[65]

## AIDS

In 1983 a group of young men in New York City with AIDS began macrobiotics under the guidance of Michio Kushi. They hoped to change their blood quality, recover their natural immunity, and survive at that time a nearly always fatal illness. In May, 1984, a research team led by Martha C. Cottrell, M.D., Director of Student Health at the Fashion Institute of Technology in New York Elinor N. Levy, Ph.D. and John C. Beldekas, Ph.D. of the Department of Immunology and Microbiology at Boston University's School of Medicine, began to monitor the blood samples and immune functions of ten men with Kaposi's sarcoma (a usual symp

tom of AIDS). They issued a series of reports on their findings. The macrobiotic approach to AIDS was outlined in *AIDS, Macrobiotics, and Natural Immunity* by Michio Kushi and Martha Cottrell, M.D., *AIDS & Diet* by Kushi and Alex Jack, and *The Way of Hope: Michio Kushi's Anti-AIDS Program* by Tom Monte.

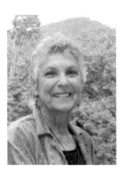

Martha C. Cottrell, M.D. led the macrobiotic AIDS project in New York

℞ **Men with AIDS Stabilize on Macrobiotics**
The NYC research team reported in *Lancet*, the British medical journal, that the men with AIDS were stabilizing on the macrobiotic diet. "Survival in these men who have received little or no medical treatment appears to compare very favorably with that of KS [Kaposi's sarcoma] patients in general. We suggest that physicians and scientists can feel comfortable in allowing patients, particularly those with minimal disease, to go untreated as part of a larger [dietary] study or because non-treatment is the patient's choice."[66]

℞ **Modern Agriculture Led to Evolution of HIV**
**In an analysis of**

In an analysis of diet and immune-defi-ciency disorders, ed-tor Michio Kushi, who led an AIDS and diet seminar for 250 medical doctors in Afri-ca sponsored by the World Health Organization (WHO), attributed the emergence of HIV and other new viruses to modern agricultural practic-es and patterns of food consumption that have disrupted traditional so-cieties and ecosystems that have existed in harmony for thousands of

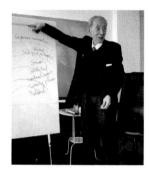

Michio Kushi led a seminar on diet and AIDS in the Republic of the Congo

years. HIV acquired its virulence and elu-siveness as a result of modern environmen-tal and medical interventions, including monocropping, pesticide and chemical ferti-lizer use, and abuse of antibiotics and other drugs. As it made its way through depleted soil, a chemically weakened food chain, and immuno-suppressed blood systems, HIV gradually evolved into a stronger, more le-thal virus. Kushi also explored the role that a modern diet based on extremely expansive foods such as sugar, sweets, fatty foods, oily and greasy foods, and fruits and juices, as well as use of too much alcohol, drugs, and medications, may have played in loss of nat-ural immunity to disease.[67]

## ☤ Umeboshi Plums Protect Against H1N1 Virus.

Umeboshi, an aged, salted, pickled plum and staple in macrobiotic cook-ing, contain a substance that can suppress the growth of the H1N1 vi-rus, researchers at the Wakayama Medical University in Japan reported. They said the substance is a type of polyphenol whose existence has not been previously confirmed. When applied to the affected cells, the growth of the virus was suppressed by roughly 90 percent after about

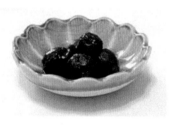

Umeboshi plums protect against infection and strengthen the blood

seven hours. "We can expect to suppress the virus growth by having about five pieces of umeboshi a day," Hirotoshi Utsunomiya, associate professor of pathology and team leader, said. Ume-Sho-Bancha and Ume-Sho-Kuzu medicinal drinks are two of the main macrobiotic home remedies for pre- venting or relieving swine flu and other infectious conditions.[68]

# Arthritis

Arthritis, a painful bone and joint disease, affects millions of people. Major forms include osteoarthritis, the painful hardening of bones and joints in the hands or spine, which affects primarily older people, especially men. Rheumatoid arthritis, involving the inflammation and swelling of the joints, especially in the hands and feet, appears primarily in women aged 25 to 50. A balanced diet has benefited many people with arthritis. In macrobiotic counseling experience, excessive animal food and salt contributes to osteoarthritis, while potatoes, tomatoes, and other nightshade plants may lead to rheumatoid arthritis.

### ⚕ Vegan Diet Improves Symptoms of Rheumatoid Arthritis

In a random case-control study of 66 patients with active rheumatoid arthritis, scientists reported that 40% of the vegan diet group experienced improvement compared to 4% of the group eating a nonvegan diet. "The immunoglobulin G (IgG) antibody levels against gliadin and beta-lactoglobulin decreased in the responder subgroup in the vegan diet-treated patients, but not in the other analysed groups." The researchers concluded that the vegan diet (which avoids all animal products and emphasizes whole grains, vegetables, and other plant quality foods) may be of benefit to certain RA patients.[69]

### ⚕ Traditional Societies Free of Arthritis

"Arthritis is not a genetic disease, nor is it an inevitable part of growing older—there are causes for these joint afflictions, and they lie in our environment—our closest contact with our environment is our food," explains Dr. John McDougall, an American holistic medical doctor. He cites research showing that rheumatoid arthritis did not exist before 1800 and that many types of arthritis were rare to nonexistent in rural regions of Africa and Asia. "As recently as 1957, no case of rheumatoid arthritis could be found in Africa. That was a time when people in Africa followed diets based on grains and vegetables." However, with the influx of meat, dairy products, and highly processed foods, arthritis began to appear in traditional societies. "An unhealthy diet containing dairy and other animal products causes inflammation of the intestinal surfaces and thereby increases the passage of dietary and/or bacterial antigens," Dr. McDougall observed.[70]

### ⚕ Nightshades Linked to Arthritis

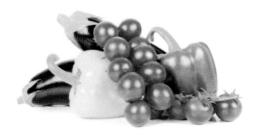

Tomatoes, potatoes, eggplant, peppers, and other members of the nightshade family are a principal cause of arthritis. In a survey of over 1400 persons over a 20-year period, researchers at Rutgers University, the University of Florida, and the Arthritis Nightshades Research Foundation reported that these plants, along with tobacco (another member of the nightshade family) are an important causative factor in arthritis in sensitive people. "Osteoarthritis appears to be a result of long-term consumption and/or use of the Solanaceae which contain naturally the active metabolite, vitamin D3, which in excess causes crippling and early disability (as seen in livestock)." Removing nightshades from the diet has "resulted in positive to marked improvement in arthritis and general health," the researchers concluded in the *Journal of Neurological and Orthopedic Medical Surgery*.[71]

## Autism

Autism, in which the child does not develop close personal relationships and lives in a world of their own, usually appears between one and three, and symptoms persist throughout life. Medically, autism is considered irreversible.

### ⚕ Sonic Rebirth

Simulating the sound of the mother's voice in utero, Alfred Tomatis, M.D., the French expert on the effects of sound and music on human development, has helped relieve many cases of autism by recreating the sound of the mother's voice in embryo and playing it back to the autistic child to reestablish the sonic contact that was disrupted in the womb. "The vocal nourishment that the mother provides is just as important as her milk," he explains. For adopted children or children whose mother isdead or incapacitated, he uses the filtered music of Mozart, which has a similar effect. Dr. Tomatis recommends a natural diet high in whole grains, fresh vegetables, and less dairy food, especially yogurt, for optimal hearing and development.[72]

### 👁 Boy Recovers from Autism with Macrobiotics and Music

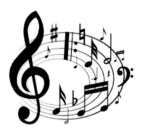

Judy and Dick Harvey adopted James, an orphan from Vietnam who was later diagnosed as autistic, in the early 1970s. The boy loved to eat french fries, cheese, candy, and salty foods, but discontinued these, along with dairy, red meat, eggs, poultry, and refined sugar following a consultation with educator Michio Kushi. Through macrobiotics and participation in classical music, he overcame his disabilities, went on to study at the University of Nebraska where he majored in math and physics, and is now living a normal life.[73]

### ☞ Autistic Girl Changes Diet and Tests Normal within a Year

After only two weeks on a macrobiotic diet, parents of an autistic little girl noticed positive changes. (The family chose to remain anonymous.) Almost daily she emerged with new skills. A year later, she was a completely different child. "Her therapists and teachers were all amazed by how much she has changed and progressed," the parents related. "When retested for speech, her scores were well above the average for her age. The only trace of autism was her pragmatic speech, and difficulty coming up with new ideas to maintain a dialog with peers. But that too was continually and rapidly improving. Incredibly, within a year she was at the level of a typically-developing child in the following ways: 1) Eye contact, 2) Joint attention, 3) the desire and initiative for social interaction and play with peers, 4) the ability to show and recognize a wide variety of emotions and appropriately respond to them, 5) pretend play skills."[74]

### ⚕ Gluten- and Dairy-Free Diets Reduce Autistic Behavior

In a review of nutritional approaches to autism, researchers at the Center for Reading Research at Stravanger University College in Norway reported that gluten and/or casein (dairy) free diets help reduce autistic behavior, increase social and communicative skills, and lead to the reappearance of autistic traits if the children go off the diet. In a randomized double-blind study of 20 autistic children, researchers in Norway found that children given a diet low in gluten, gliadin, and casein (dairy protein) developed significantly better than controls.[75]

## Celiac Disease

Celiac disease (DC) is a genetic disorder of the small intestine. Exposure to wheat, barley, rye, and other gluten products causes an inflammatory response that atrophies the villi and interferes with absorption. CD was first described in the 1880s and linked to wheat only in the 1940s. While the disorder is hard to reverse, a macrobiotic way of eating, centered on rice, millet, and other non-glutenous grains, usually improves digestion. *See Gluten Sensitivity below.*

### ☞ Refining of Wheat May Underlie Celiac

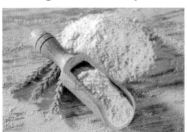

For thousands of years, wheat, barley, and other glutinous foods were consumed as staple foods without any reported intolerances or digestive problems. The emergence of Celiac in the late 19th century accompanied the refining of grains that made cheap white bread widely available. According to macrobiotic researcher Alex Jack, consumption of excessive refined flour and other adulterated gluten products may have led to a gene mutation that was inheritable among susceptible family members. A similar process appears to have led to the mutation of the BRCA gene linked to breast cancer following increased dairy consumption in Europe. In the case of Celiac, the villi of the small intestine appear to have lost the ability to function properly after excessive exposure to refined flour, especially that made with commercial baker's yeast and other additives.[76]

## Children's Health

Nutritionists and physicians initially raised questions about the adequacy of the macrobiotic regimen for children, especially since they were not getting dairy products. But over the years, scientific and medical studies generally found that macrobiotic youngsters were adequately nourished and, in many cases, exceeded the nutritional levels of ordinary children eating the modern way.

### ⚕ Macrobiotic Day-Care Center a Model for British Children

A British nutritionist found that a macrobiotic day-care center in London not only "supported normal growth" in nursery school children but also could be used as a model to implement national dietary guidelines. Comparing the nutritional adequacy of macrobiotic meals provided pre-school children by the Community Health Foundation with ordinary meals at a nursery in Notting Hill, the investigator found that the macro-biotic food met current U.K.-R.D.I. dietary, energy, and nutrient standards and that the children's anthropometric measurements including weight, height, and skinfold thicknesses were normal. In contrast, the ordinary nursery school diet was high in dairy food, lard, and other saturated fats that have been associated with the development of atherosclerosis beginning in childhood. "This illustrates the power and potential of nursery meals to contribute to the adoption of a nutritionally sound and beneficial national diet."[77]

### ⚕ Macrobiotic Children Develop Normally

In a study of vegetarian preschool children, researchers at New England Medical Center Hospital in Boston found that the growth of macrobiotic youngsters did not significantly differ from those of non-macrobiotics before age two. After age two, macrobiotic children tended to put on weight more quickly than the chil-dren brought up on yoga diets, Seventh-Day Adventist diets, or other vegetarian regimes. Nearly all the children had been breast-fed, and it was found that macrobiotic children who had been weaned did not differ in caloric intake from non-macrobiotics, according to the study published in *Pediatrics*.[78]

### ⚕ Macrobiotic Children Have Higher IQs

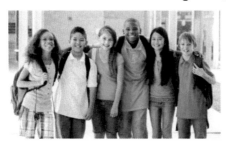

In a study of mental development, macrobiotic and vegetarian children were brighter and more intelligent than ordinary youngsters their age. The mean I.Q. was 116 for the group as a whole, or 16 percent above average.

**Macrobiotic children test healthy and have higher IQs than other kids**

The children's mean mental age was found to exceed their mean chronologic age by approximately a year. The macrobiotic children's I.Q.'s and mental ages were slightly higher than the other vegetarians. "In the judgments of both the pediatrician and psychologic technician, the children as a group were bright," the researchers concluded in the *Journal of the Amercian Dietetic Association*. They speculated, however, that the brightness may be due to better education on the part of the macrobiotic and vegetarian parents, not to diet.[79]

## Crohn's Disease

Crohn's Disease is an inflammatory bowel disease for which there is no medical cure. However, it lends itself to improvement or recovery with a macrobiotic diet.

### ⚕ Free of Crohn's for 35 Years

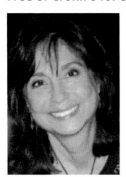

After suffering for seven years from Crohn's, Virginia Harper recovered with the help of macrobiotics. Over the last 35 years, she has enjoyed optimal health and gone on to become a leading macrobiotic teacher and counselor. At You Can Heal You, her healing center in Nashville, Virginia has helped many others with digestive disorders and teaches worldwide. She is the author of *Controlling Crohn's the Natural Way*.[80]

**After recovering, Virginia Harper guided many others to greater health**

## Diabetes

Nearly 30 million Americans—1 in 8—are diagnosed with diabetes, the fastest growing chronic disease in the country, and nearly 300 million people around the globe have the condition. According to the World Health Organization (WHO), the number of cases will double by 2030. Special programs on a dietary approach to diabetes were offered at Kushi Institute and other macrobiotic centers. In Italy, the International Un Punto Macrobiotico Foundation sponsored diabetes intervention studies in Thailand, Cuba, and other countries. Planetary Health, Inc. proposed a macrobiotic study for the Middle East, where diabetes is skyrocketing, and published a primer *Diabetes: The Macrobiotic Approach*.

### ⚕ Thai Patients Get Off Insulin on Macrobiotic Diet

A study by the Ministry of Public Health in Thailand found that a macrobiotic way of eating (known as the Ma-Pi 2 Diet) designed by Italian educator Mario Pianesi offers an effective, alternate approach to the care of diabetes patients and that it may help patients on insulin maintain their blood sugar levels without an insulin injection. In a dietary intervention study at the Wanakaset Research Facility of Kasetart University in Trad Province, researchers found a statistically significant reduction in blood sugar levels, weight, blood pressure, and heartbeat ratios among 44 patients put on a macrobiotic way of eating. "Subjects were in significantly better health, more vibrant, more peaceful, and more energetic," the study reported in 2006. The four patients on insulin were able to maintain their blood sugar levels within the range of 110-171 mg without any insulin injections and all subjects were free of any adverse effects.[81]

### ⚕ Cuban Patients Get Off Insulin

In a 6-month macrobiotic dietary intervention study of the Ma-Pi 2 Diet carried out in 16 adults with Type 2 diabetes at the Diabetic Care Center in Colon, Cuban physicians reported in 2009 that anthropometric variables significantly improved, including lean body mass and glucide and lipid metabolism. "All participants were able to eliminate insulin treatment, and 25 percent continued treatment with glibenclamide only," the researchers reported. "According to lipid levels and ratios, cardiovascular risk was also considerably reduced." The investigators noted. "Hemoglobin, total protein, albumin, and creatinin levels indicated that nutritional safety was maintained. There were no adverse events."[82]

### ⚕ Brown Rice Reduces Diabetes Risk

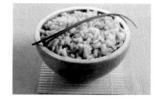

Researchers from the Harvard School of Public Health (HSPH) have found that eating five or more servings of white rice per week was associated with an increased risk oftype 2 diabetes. In contrast, eating two or more servings of brown rice per week was associated with a lower risk of the disease. The researchers estimated that replacing 50 grams of white rice (just one third of a typical daily serving) with the same amount of brown rice would lower risk of type 2 diabetes by 16%. The same replacement with other whole grains was associated with a 36% reduced risk.[83]

### ⚕ American Patients Get Off or Reduce Insulin
In a review of the macrobiotic approach to diabetes, Robert H. Lerman, M.D., Ph.D. cited a recent case series in 13 patients with type 2 diabetes provided with nutrition education and provided with meals at the Kushi Institute. Under the supervision of Margaret Cottrell, M.D., most experienced reduction in or elimination of diabetes medication, weight loss, reduced blood pressure, and improvement in energy after starting the new way of eating in the course of the program.[84]

### ⚕ Macrobiotics Shows Most Improved Glycemic Control
In a systematic review of dietary patterns and management of type 2 diabetes, Australian researchers found that "mounting evidence supports the view that vegan vegetarian, and Mediterranean dietary patterns should be implemented in public health strategies, in order to better control glycemic markers in individuals with T2DM. They found that the macrobiotic diet showed the most improved glycemic control among the plant-based diets reviewed.[85]

## Ebola
Following the outbreak of Ebola in 2014, the macrobiotic community prepared dietary guidelines for the epidemic then raging in West Africa.

### ⌕ Modern Agriculture Linked to New Viral Diseases

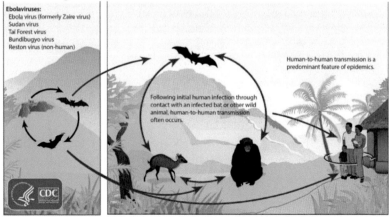

In consultation with Michio Kushi, Planetary Health researchers Alex Jack, Edward Esko, and Sachi Kato hypothesized that Ebola broke out in Central Africa following the introduction of monoculture and commodity crops, especially cassava and bananas, which displaced grains, beans, and other organic and natural crops. The changes upset the delicate checks and balances in the soil biota and in local ecosystems, giving rise to virulent new strains of microorganisms. After coming into contact with chimpanzees or other primates infected with Ebola virus, SIV (Simian Immune-deficiency Virus, the precursor to HIV), and other pathogens or eating contaminated bushmeat, people in this region acquired natural immune deficiency, and Marburg (1967), Ebola (1976), AIDS (1981), and other lethal diseases took hold and spread. In the case of Ebola, the virus originated with contaminated fruit that was eaten by bats and passed to primates and humans. The potency of the virus increased with each mammal and compounded its virulence. The guidelines, including home remedies to treat symptoms, appeared on **www.ebolaanddiet.com** and helped airlines personnel, travelers, and others in the region deal with the emergency.[86]

## Environmental Illness

Macrobiotics has been helpful in dealing with environmental illness and chemical sensitivity.

### ♆ Physician Heals E.I. with Macrobiotic Diet

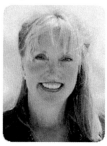

Sherry Rodger, M.D. used diet to recover from severe chemical sensitivities

In 1974 Sherry A. Rogers, M.D., a 31-year-old physician, suffered from Environmental Illness. She had ugly red eczema over the lower half of her face, periodic asthma, recurrent sinus problems, wicked migraines, chronic back pain from an old riding injury, and unwarranted exhaustion and depression. By the early 1980s she was having strong adverse reactions to chemicals such as workmen gluing down a new Formica countertop. She had treated her sensitivities with injections, multiple vitamins and ionizers, cotton blankets and pillows, bottled water, oxygen tanks, aluminum foil. In 1987, after following a macrobiotic diet for six months, the excruciating shoulder pain disappeared, and over the next few months other chronic symptoms vanished.[87]

### ⚕ Diet Helps Patients Suffering from Chemical Sensitivity

In a study of 160 patients suffering from chemical sensitivity, those who followed a macrobiotic diet for at least one year reported an average decrease in chemical sensitivity of 76 percent, according to an article in the *Journal of Applied Nutrition*.[88]

## Geriatrics

The term "macrobiotics" means long life, and a balanced, whole foods diet has traditionally been associated with healthy aging and prolonging life. In one study in at a Boston hospital, researchers found that geriatric patients experienced significant improvement on a macrobiotic diet.

### ⚕ Macrobiotics Assists Psychiatric and Geriatric Patients

Dr. Jonathan Lieff, Chief of Psychiatry and Geriatric Services at the Shattuck Hospital in Boston and doctors at Tufts University School of Nutrition, designed an experiment in 1982 to test the effect of macrobiotic food on long-term psychiatric and geriatric patients. Some of these people had been confined in the hospital for 30 years or more. In a double-blind study in which neither the ordinary hospital staff or patients knew they were participating, macrobiotic meals avoiding meat, sugar, processed foods, and synthetic food additives and including whole grains, legumes, fresh vegetables and fruits designed to look and taste like regular foods were introduced to a ward of 16 patients over an eight-week period and 18 controls. Altogether 187 food items on the macrobiotic menu were prepared, as well as chicken, coffee, and butter which were difficult to simulate. During the test, the researchers noted medically significant reductions in psychosis and agitation among the patients. The scientists found significant improvement in experimental group cooperativeness when compared to the control group, as well as less irritability and improvement upon manifest psychosis. "These data show that the described change in total diet does have a significantly favorable effect on the health and behavior of geropsychiatric patients," the observers concluded.[89]

## Gluten Intolerance

Celiac affects only a tiny fraction of the population, while gluten intolerance affects millions of people. It arose following the introduction of new hybrid varieties of dwarf wheat during the Green Revolution in the 1950s and 1960s. The wheat led to higher yields but required synthetic fertilizers and pesticides and much more water. When switching to organic whole wheat or barley from heirloom seeds, many people with gluten sensitivities are able to digest gluten without difficulty. Macrobiotics has been helpful for many people with gluten sensitivities.[90]

### Ex-Gluten Sufferer Changes Diet and Enthuses 'I Love Gluten'

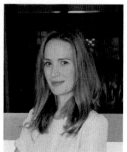

Born in Russia, Katya Thomas moved to the Netherlands with her family while she was a teenager. By her early twenties, she had developed severe gluten allergies. Just the taste of a morsel of food containing wheat, barley, or oats would precipitate violent symptoms. Doctors told her that she would have to avoid glutinous products the rest of her life. But on a gluten-free diet, Katya soon discovered that most of the products targeted for people like her contained sugar, chemicals, and other ingredients that only made her condition worse. Determined to heal herself naturally, Katya tried many vegetarian and vegan approaches. Ultimately, a balanced macrobiotic

**Katya Thomas recovered from gluten intolerance and is now a natural foods cook and healer**

diet not only regularized her digestion, but also enabled her to enjoy wheat and other glutenous foods again. Today she is a natural foods cook, consultant, and healer, and her story "I Love Gluten" and classes have helped others recover from gluten sensitivities.[91]

## Hospital Food

The modern hospital diet dates to Fanny Farmer, the popular cookbook author who was the first woman to lecture at Harvard Medical School in the early 20th century. Her medicinal recipes were as bland and tasteless as her ordinary recipes were rich and artery-clogging. Macrobiotics has been introduced into several hospitals and influenced many others to begin to serve whole grains, fresh foods, and other healing foods.

### Boston Hospital Serves Macrobiotic Food

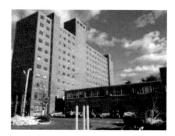

In 1980, a macrobiotic lunch program was started at the Lemuel Shattuck Hospital in Boston for doctors, nurses, and staff. Overall response was favorable and improved noticeably after the macrobiotic food line was integrated with the regular cafeteria line. By the second year, half of the food served each day in the cafeteria was prepared macrobiotically. Regular attendance inCreased from about 60 to 120 to 200 persons each day. At lunch, from 70 to

**Shattuck Hospital instituted a macrobiotic lunch program**

90 percent of all meals served included at least one item from the macrobiotic menu. Dr. William Castelli, director of the Framingham Heart Study, contrasted the healthfulness of the macrobiotic food program at the Shattuck Hospital with ordinary hospital food.[92]

### ⚕ Irish Hospital Offers Macrobiotic Meals

Macrobiotic food was introduced at the National Children's Hospital in Dublin, Ireland. Cecilia Armelin, pediatric dietitian, drew up a sample meal plan including for breakfast: whole oat porridge; for lunch: miso soup with dulse and parsley, brown rice with haricot or azuki beans, Brussels sprouts, dried apricots and raisins; and for dinner: lentil/barley soup seasoned with miso and parsley and whole grain millet with pears and chopped walnuts. She especially recommended these foods for children with multiple allergies or food intolerance.[93]

## Longevity

### ⚕ Macrobiotic Oriented Diet Promotes Longevity

In a study of mortality from all causes, public health researchers in Vienna reported that a high intake of whole grains, vegetables, fruits, nuts, and coffee is associated with a reduced risk for all-causes of death whereas a high intake of red meat and especially processed meat is positively related to all-cause mortality.[94]

## Medical Education

Until recently, medical schools offered little if any instruction in nutrition. As alternative medicine went mainstream, they began to encourage their students to become familiar with acupuncture, macrobiotics, yoga, and other popular complementary approaches.

### ⚕ AMA Encourages Students to Sample Macrobiotic Meal

By 1998, the American Medical Association reported that two-thirds of medical schools in the United States were offering courses in alternative and complementary medicine. Among the key recommendations offered by the physicians was that the new medical school curricula include an experiential component. Macrobiotics was singled out in *JAMA* (*Journal of the American Medical Association*) as one of the principal modalities which young medical school students should be familiar with: "Experiencing acupuncture or therapeutic massage or tasting a macrobiotic meal adds a dimension to the learning experience that a lecture or simple demonstration cannot. The deeper understanding that results should provide a better basis for responsibly advising patients."[95]

By 2015, nearly 90% offered courses in alternative medicine, according to the Association of American Medical Colleges.[96]

## Mental and Emotional Health

From the macrobiotic view, there is no rigid distinction between mind and body and between spirit and matter. Food governs mental, emotional, and spiritual health as well as physical health and vitality. Individuals and families have come a variety of mental and emotional conditions ranging from anxiety and depression to schizophrenia and other severe mental illnesses.

### Man Recovers from Schizophrenia with Macrobiotics

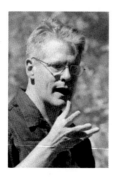

David Briscoe became a leading teacher

With the help of his mother, Charlotte Mahoney-Briscoe, David Briscoe healed himself of schizophrenia by adhering to a balanced macrobiotic diet. David, diagnosed with mental and emotional illness in the 1960s, unsuccessfully tried many hospitals, medications, and confinement before changing his diet. In high school, he become physically ill, with acute kidney problems, frequent sore throats, digestive problems, fevers, and a duodenal ulcer. For his depression, he went to psychiatrists for six years and became addicted to Thorazine. After changing his way of eating to brown rice, soy sauce, and other foods, he made a complete recovery. David is currently married, the father of four children, and director of Macrobiotics America, an online school.[97]

### Diet Effective in Treating Mental Illness

Dr. Stephen Harnish, a New Hampshire psychiatrist, reported that macrobiotics had benefited many of his patients who were chronically and severely mentally ill. Citing several case histories, he described a young woman with a history of severe depression who had been in a state hospital for two years and treated with anti-depressants and antipsychotic medications. Tests by Dr. Harnish's department found that the woman was hypoglycemic and administration of a macrobiotic diet high in complex carbohydrates and one that avoided animal food and sugar resulted in steady improvement, reduced medication, and return to normal functioning. "She now has motivation to do new things and has made plans to return to school." He noted that hundreds of other psychiatric patients could benefit from this approach.[98]

## Microwave Cooking

A clean, natural flame is ideal for cooking. Wood, gas, kerosen or other renewable energy source is best. Macrobiotics discoura microwave cooking that give a chaotic vibration and weaken the

### ⚕ Microwaved Food Alters Blood Chemistry

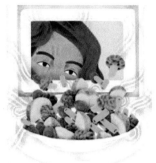

In a study of people eating a macrobiotic diet, researchers at the Swiss Institute of Technology and the University for Biochemistry and the Environmental-Biological Research and Consultation reported that microwaved food produced a decrease in hemoglobin; an increase in hematocrit, and leukocytes; higher cholesterol, and a decrease in lymphocytes. In addition to altering blood chemistry, the researchers found that microwaved food appeared to increase the activity of certain bacteria in the food, and altered cells resembled the pathogenic stages that occur in the early development of some cancers. The scientists also reported biological changes in the microwaved food itself, including increased acidity, damaged protein molecules, enlarged fat cells, and decreased folic acid, a nutrient in the vitamin B group associated with protecting against spina bifida, a birth defect.[99]

## Migraine and PMS

Over the years, the East West Foundation, Kushi Institute, and other macrobiotic organizations published case histories of of people who recovered from scores of common conditions ranging from flu and infectious diseases to female disorders, from digestive and circulatory conditions to severe nervous disorders.

### ⚕ Severe Headaches and Female Complaints Eliminated

A former medical consultant for the Department of National Health and Welfare in Canada successfully treated her own migraine headaches with a macrobiotic diet. Dr. Helen V. Farrell reported that she suffered from classical migraines since she was eleven, experiencing scintillating scotomas, dysplasia, transient parasthesias, and vomiting. As she grew older, the headaches were less frequent, and when she discontinued dairy food and exercised regularly they began to disappear altogether. Dr. Farrell, who specializes in treating female complaints, has successfully introduced many of her patients to a macrobiotic diet. She reports that it is particularly effective in treating premenstrual syndrome.[100]

### ⚕ Plant-Based Diet Improves Symptoms of Multiple Sclerosis

In a modified dietary intervention study for 128 women with multiple sclerosis, medical researchers in the United States put subjects on a diet high in whole grains, vegetables, fresh fruits, and fish and other foods high in poly- and monounsaturated fats. Meat, dairy, and most processed foods were eliminated, and salt intake limited. The scientists reported "reduced fatigue, impact of MS symptoms, and disability." Compliance in the study was extremely high during the year: 94.4%.[101]

## Nuclear Radiation

From the atomic bombings of Hiroshima and Nagasaki to nuclear accidents in the Soviet Union, macrobiotic quality foods proved instrumental in preventing and relieving atomic sickness, including leukemia, thyroid cancer, and other consequences of excessive exposure to radioactivity. Medical studies in Japan and Canada confirmed the ability of miso and sea vegetables to discharge Cesium-37, Strontium-90, and other radioactive particles from the body. In 1990, the Kushi Institute organized an airlift of thousands of pounds of miso, seaweed, and other major staples to give to Soviet medical doctors in Chelyabinsk and Chernobyl.

### ⚕ Macrobiotic Diet Saves All Patients in Nagasaki

In August, 1945, at the time of the atomic bombing of Japan, Tatsuichiro Akizuki, M.D., was director of the Department of Internal Medicine at St. Francis's Hospital in Nagasaki. Most patients in the hospital, located one mile from the center of the blast, survived the initial effects of the bomb, but soon after came down with symptoms of radiation sickness from the fallout that had been released. Dr. Akizuki fed his staff and patients a strict macrobiotic diet of brown rice, miso soup, wakame and other sea vegeta-

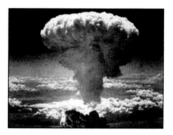

**All patients at St. Francis Hospital in Nagasaki survived atomic sickness on a macrobiotic diet**

bles, Hokkaido pumpkin, and sea salt and prohibited the consumption of sugar and sweets. As a result, he saved everyone in his hospital, while many other survivors in the city perished from radiation sickness. "I gave the cooks and staff strict orders that they should make unpolished whole-grain rice balls, adding some salt to them, prepare strong miso soup for each meal, and never use sugar. When they didn't follow my orders, I scolded them without mercy, 'Never take sugar. Sugar will destroy your blood!'. . ."This dietary method made it possible for me to remain alive and go on working vigorously as a doctor. . . . It was thanks to this food that all of us could work for people day after day, overcoming fatigue or symptoms of atomic disease and survive the disaster free from severe symptoms of radioactivity."[102]

## Miso Soup Key Food in Protecting Against Nuclear Fallout

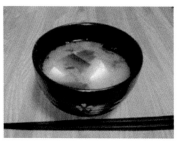

Atomic bomb survivors credited miso with helping to prevent radiation sickness .

In interviews sixty years after the atomic bombing of Japan, seven former patients at St. Francis Hospital, fourteen other atomic survivors in Nagasaki, and eight survivors in Hiroshima described how miso soup and other macrobiotic quality foods helped them prevent or relieve radiation sickness. Analyzing her findings, Hiroko Furo, an associate professor at Illinois Wesleyan University, concluded that "miso was very helpful for the survivors' healing and that macrobiotic food contributed to the easing atomic bomb syndrome." Dr. Furo suggested that the macrobiotic diet would be useful for those who are undergoing radiation therapy and may eventually be incorporated into the medical treatment of cancer.[103]

## Kelp Protects Against Nuclear Fallout and Radiation

During the Cold War, scientists at the Gastro-Intestinal Research Laboratory at McGill University in Montreal, Canada, reported that a substance derived from the sea vegetable kelp could reduce by 50 to 80 percent the amount of radioactive strontium absorbed through the intestine. Stanley Skoryna, M.D. said in the *Canadian Medical Journal* in 1964 that in animal experiments sodium alginate obtained from brown algae permitted calcium to be normally absorbed through the intestinal wall while binding most of the strontium. The sodium alginate and strontium were subsequently excreted from the body. The experiments were designed to devise a method to counteract the effects of fallout and radiation.[104]

## Miso Eliminates Deadly Iodine-131 from the Body

Following up the macrobiotic survivals in Hiroshima and Nagasaki from radition sickness at the end of World War II, Japanese reseachers reported that miso is effective in helping to remove radioactive elements from the body and controlling inflammation of organs caused by radioactivity. In laboratory studies, researchers at Hiroshima

University Medical Center found that there was only half the amount of radioactive iodine 131 in the blood of the group of rats fed with miso in contrast to the control group three and six hours after the injections. Lower amounts of radioactive particles were also measured in the kidneys, liver, and spleen. Although there was no difference in the amount of radioactive cesium in the blood, a high amount of cesium was eliminated from the muscles of the group eating miso.[105]

## ☤ Macrobiotic Diet Helps Victims of Soviet Nuclear Accidents

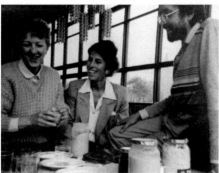

Soviet physicians Lidia Yamchuk (left) and Hanif Shaimardanov (right) used macrobiotics to help heal victims of nuclear accidents. Macrobiotic teacher Cary Wolf, part of a delegation from the Kushi Institute in America that donated thousands of pounds of miso, sea vegetables, and other natural foods, is in the center

Lidia Yamchuk and Hanif Shaimardanov, medical doctors in Cheljabinsk, organized Longevity, the first macrobiotic association in the Soviet Union in 1985. At their hospital, they used dietary methods and acupuncture to treat many patients, especially those suffering from leukemia, lymphoma, and other disorders associated with exposure to nuclear radiation. Since the early 1950s, wastes from Soviet weapons production were dumped into Karachay Lake in Cheljabinsk, an industrial city about 900 miles east of Moscow that was the center for Soviet nuclear weapons production during the Cold War. In Leningrad, Yuri Stavitsky, a young pathologist and medical instructor, volunteered as a radiologist in Chernobyl after the nuclear accident on April 26, 1986. Since then, like many disaster workers, he suffered symptoms associated with radiation disease, including tumors of the thyroid. "Since beginning macrobiotics," he reported, "my condition has greatly improved."[106]

## Obesity

Two out of three American adults and one out of three children are overweight or obese.  These  are  major risk factors for diabetes, heart disease, selected cancers, and other disorders. Almost everyone who starts macrobiotics loses weight as green protein and polyunsaturated fats and oils replace animal-quality protein and saturated fat. The Kushi Institute instituted a popular Weight-Loss Seminar and macrobiotic counselors and personal chefs were consulted frequently for this condition.

### ⚕ Kanten Key Food in Weight Loss Diet

Kanten, the traditional Japanese gelatin, made from agar-agar seaweed and an important part of the macrobiotic way of eating, is a key food to reduce obesity and chronic disease. In a study of 76 overweight patients given a balanced weight-loss diet, Japanese scientists report that those given a small serving of kanten before their dinner lost 4.4 percent of

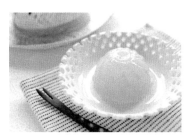

Kanten, a plant-based gelatin, assists in weight loss

their body weight over 12 weeks compared to 2.2 percent by controls.[107]

## Osteoporosis

Osteoporosis, the thinning of the bones and susceptibility to fracture, commonly occurs in middle aged and elderly people as a result of eating too much meat, dairy food, and other animal protein that leech calcium and other minerals from the bones, as well as excessive salt, caffeine, alcohol, and smoking. In addition to avoiding or reducing these foods, natto is particularly effective in treating this affliction. Natto, fermented soybeans that clump together with long sticky strands, has been a staple in Far Eastern cooking and macrobiotic healthcare. It is especially beneficial for the intestines and digestion.

### ⚕ Natto Helps Relieve Osteoporosis

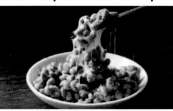

Natto, fermented soybeans, protect against bone loss

In a study on the effect of consuming natto on bone density, Japanese scientists found that total hipbone mineral density increased with increasing habitual natto intake in postmenopausal women, although not at other skeletal sites. There was also improvement at the femoral neck and at the radius in older women.[108] Natto's antibiotic and antitumor properties are now being investigated. It is also effective in reducing the effects of hangovers.

## Pregnancy and Childbirth

The Kushis had five children, wrote *Raising Healthy Kids* and *Macrobiotic Pregnancy and Care of the Newborn* with Edward and Wendy Esko, longtime macro biotic teachers and parents of eight children, and gave many seminars on children's and family health. As a rule, they recommended natural home birth or assistance of a midwife in a hospital setting. In many cases, dietary modification or adjustment would successfully deal with any problems encountered. However, for difficult deliveries, they sometimes recommended acupuncture, moxibustion (burning herbs to stimulate acupuncture points), or shiatsu massage. Prayer and meditation are also important healing methods they encouraged. At the Kushi Institute, the One Peaceful World Children's Shrine and Memorial was erected to honor the spirits of unborn children who died prematurely through abortion, miscarriage, accident, or disease. Modern medicine has validated the use of traditional Far Eastern methods for assisting childbirth.

### 🕈 Moxibustion Aids Breech Births

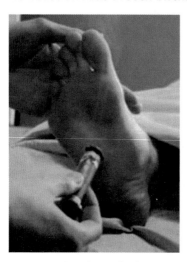

Moxa, or burning an herb on an acupressure point is effective for difficulty deliveries and many other conditions

In China, moxibustion (burning herbs to stimulate acupuncture points) was traditionally used to treat breech babies. In a study designed to evaluate the efficacy and safety of moxa, researchers at the Women's Hospital of Jiangxi Province, Nanchang, and Jiujiang Women's and Children's Hospital devised a clinical trial of 260 expectant mothers with breech presentation. The women were randomly divided into two groups. During the thirty-third week of pregnancy, the intervention group received stimulation of acupoint BL 67 (on the bladder meridian on the outside corner of the fifth toenail) for seven days with treatment for an additional seven days if necessary. Fetal movement correlated with overall success in righting the developing babies. The intervention group experienced an average of 48 fetal movements vs 35 in the control group and although 24 subjects in the control group and 1 in the intervention group underwent external cephalic version, 98 of the 130 fetuses in the intervention group were cephalic at birth vs 81 in the control group of 130 fetuses. The findings were published in the *Journal of the American Medical Association* and lauded by the AMA.[109]

### ⚕ Moxa and Acupuncture May Reduce Caesarean Section

In a review of six trials of the traditional Chinese use of moxa for breech deliveries, researchers concluded, "There is some evidence to suggest that the use of moxibustion may reduce the need for oxytocin. When combined with acupuncture, moxibustion may result in fewer births by caesarean section; and when combined with postural management techniques may reduce the number of non-cephalic presentations at birth."[110]

### ⚕ Shiatsu and Acupuncture Aid Childbirth

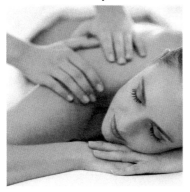

Shiatsu massage is relaxing and stimulates Ki energy flow.

According to Chinese medicine, a correct balance of Qi (life energy) and quantity of blood are vital in order to commence labor and continue the childbirth process. Correspondingly, there are two main reasons for a delayed or difficult childbirth: lack of Qi and blood or stagnation of Qi and blood. In a retrospective study of 80 women aged 22-40 who required labor inducement, researchers compared traditional inducement methods (including shiatsu and/or acupuncture), conventional methods (pharmaceutical, mechanical), and a combination of both. Researchers found that traditional inducement methods, whether or not combined with conventional methods, are an important and effective tool in their ability to reduce the extent of intervention throughout the birth process and also in reducing delivery completion interventions. "Significant difference was found in shortening labor process when inducement treatment combined both Chinese medicine and conventional methods, in comparison to conventional inducement alone {medicinal/mechanical)," the researchers concluded. "This is an important result considering the high availability and low cost of Chinese treatment, and especially because it is a non-harmful method of inducement."[111]

# Lifestyle

## Chewing

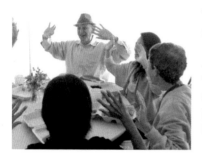

Thorough chewing benefits mind, body, and spirit. In a review of chewing and its effects, including many scientific and medical studies and personal accounts, two macrobiotic teachers and counselors conclude that proper chewing (approximately 50 or more times per mouthful) contributes to health at many levels:

**Marathon chewer Lino Stanchich leads a lunchtime discussion**

- **Proper Digestion** Chewing protects against hunger, starvation, and disease and is essential for proper digestion; contributes to health and vitality, and prolongs life. It charges the food, activating the entire organism
- **Improves Taste of Food** Chewing improves the sensory qualities of food. It makes grains sweeter to the taste, stimulates the appetite, and contributes to greater awareness of texture, smell, and aroma
- **Stabilizes the Emotions** Chewing helps stabilize the emotions and by slowing down consumption and improving taste contributes to the aesthetic enjoyment of the meal
- **Calms the Mind** Chewing calms the mind, strengthens the intellect, and contributes to greater clarity, insight, and understanding
- **Reduces Food Waste** Chewing contributes to greater harmony within the family, in society, and with the environment, including better communication with others, increased awareness of earth and sky, and less use of energy and waste of food (including packaging materials, transport, and disposal)
- **Enhances Spiritual Awareness** Chewing contributes to spiritual awareness, including deeper knowledge of the order of nature and the universe, stronger intuition, and discovery of one's dream in life
- **Contributes to Universal Consciousness** Chewing contributes to universal awareness, including the free play of consciousness on all levels and oneness with all of life

In addition to examining the physiology of digestion, the study describes the traditional use of saliva for healing, especially by Jesus and Mohammad.[112]

## Exercise and Fitness

Exercise, fitness, and physical activity are an important dimension of daily health. Eating a balanced, grain-centered diet can also translated into winning on the ball field.

### ✍ Macrobiotic Japanese Baseball Team Wins Championship

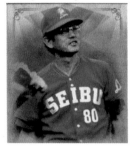

In 1983, a Japanese professional baseball team climbed from last to first place by switching to a macrobiotic diet. After taking over the last place Seibu Lions in October, 1981, manager Tatsuro Hirooka initiated a dietary experiment. Restricting the players' intake of meat, sugar, and white rice, he encouraged them to eat brown rice, tofu, vegetables, and soybean products. He told the players that animal food increases an athlete's susceptibility to injuries. Conversely, natural foods, they were told, protect the body from sprains and dislocation

The Seibu Lions defeated the Ham-Fighters.

keep the mind clear and focused. During the 1982 season, the Lions were ridiculed by their archrivals, the Nippon Ham Fighters, a team sponsored by a major meat company. However, the Lions defeated the Ham-Fighters for the Pacific League crown and continued to the Japan World Series and beat the Chunichi Dragons. The Lions won the championship again the following year as well.[113]

## Arts and Culture

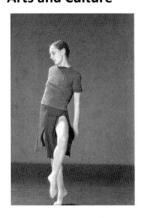

Dancer Anne Teresa de Keersmacher

Many singers, dancers, and movie stars have observed a macrobiotic way or employed macrobiotic chefs, including Gloria Swanson, Maurice Cunningham, Madonna, Sting, Anne Teresa de Keeermacher, Demi Moore, Pamela Anderson, Gwyneth Paltrow, Alicia Silverstone, Fiona Apple, Nicole Kidman, Tom Cruise, and John Travolta. As singer John Denver enthused, "On a macrobiotic diet, I had all the energy in the world, clear-headed and singing like a bird! I loved it, I felt great!" In addition to a healthy glow, improved vitality, a trimmer physique, and greater flexibility, some performers also use macrobiotic principles:

- **Composer John Cage** John Cage whom *Time* hailed as "the puckish composer, audacious theoretician, stylish writer, subtle graphic artist, macrobiotic guru and fearless mushroom hunter . . . the impish personification of the 20th century avant-garde" used the I Ching and Far Eastern principles to compose music. His colleague dancer Maurice Cunningham was also macrobiotic.[114]
- **Artist Rod House** Rod House, one of Michio Kushi's earliest students, taught at the New England College of Art, and was on the original faculty of the Kushi Institute. His paintings have been exhibited throughout New England.
- **Painter and Sculptor Patricia Price** Patricia Price, an English artist and painter, taught art at the Kushi Institute and sculpted a large Jizo Bodhisattva.
- **Dancer and Choreographer Anne Teresa de Keersmacher** Founder, director, and choreographer of Rosas Dance Company in Brussels, Anne Teresa uses yin and yang, the five transformations, and other macrobiotic principles in her compositions. Her company performs worldwide, e.g., staging spiral dances at the Museum of Modern Art (MoMA) in New York, and her dance school has a macrobiotic dining room.

# Social Health

## Ancient Food Pattern

Since the time of Darwin and the introduction of evolutionary theory, scientists believed that meat eating was largely responsible for the development of human prowess, intellect, and ingenuity. Over the last generation, a revolution in anthropology, archaeology, and other social sciences has led to an emerging view that ancient hominins were not primarily hunters, but gatherers, and that plant-based foods largely shaped and influenced our unique human qualities.

### Present Day Hunter-Gatherers Eat Mostly Plants
Contemporary hunter-gather societies such as the Son and Kalahari bushmen in Africa consume the vast majority of their food in the form of foraged plants, fruits, and nuts and only small amounts, 10-20%, in the form of animal food.[115]

### Evidence of Plant-Based Diets Doesn't Survive Well
"The archaeological evidence [for plant-eating] is especially weak, as many organic materials, especially plants, do not survive well, and are therefore invisible in the archaeological record," the *European Journal of Clinical Nutrition* reported in 2002. Artifacts, such as stone tools which are likely to be used for hunting and animal bones with evidence of hu-

man processing and butchering do indicate that hunting did occur at many times in the past, but it is impossible to judge the frequency."[116]

## ⚕ Cooking Made Us Human

In *Catching Fire: How Cooking Made Us Human,* Harvard primatologist Richard Wrangham hypothesized that the mastery of fire for cooking spurred the development of early humans, not meat-eating. Cooking, in his view, made more calories from existing, largely plant quality foods, available and improved metabolism, leading to the development of larger brains. Cooking also facilitated warmth, leading to the loss of body hair and the ability to run faster without overheating. Wrangham suggests it also allowed early hominins to develop more peaceful personalities, develop new social structures around the hearth, and bring the sexes closer together. Raw food, he contends, does not supply enough caloric energy and is unsustainable and can cause up to half the women to cease menstruation. Cooking increases the net energy gain by 30%.[117] As humans evolved from the monkey and primate state, they discovered cycles of change, found ways to store food, and learned to cook. As a result of his investigations, Wrangham became vegetarian.

## ⚕ Wild Grasses as Principal Food

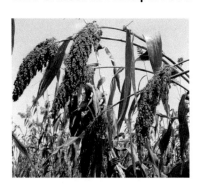

**Sorghum was the ancestral grain of the earliest humans in Africa**

In the early twenty-first century, evidence started to emerge that *homo sapiens* ate wild grasses, the prototype of grains, as principal food. At the University of Colorado Boulder researchers reported: "High tech tests on tooth enamel by researchers indicate that prior to about 4 million year ago, Africa's hominids were eating essentially chimpanzee style, dining on fruits and some leaves," explained anthropology professor Matt Sponheimer, lead author of the 2013 study. "A new look at the diets of ancient African hominids shows a 'game change' occurred about 3.5 million years ago when some members added grasses or sedges (a family of rushes including water chestnut) to their menus."[118] "It is quite possible that these changes in diet were an important step in becoming human," he concluded.

### Lucy, Mother of Humankind, a Vegetarian

For nearly 2 million years, *Australopithecus,* the primary hominin ancestors in Africa, was largely vegetarian. *Australopithecus anamensis,* a hominid that lived in East Africa more than 4 millions years ago, was herbivorous. Lucy, often referred to as the Eve or mother of the human race, lived about a million years later. Her skeletal remains, found in East Africa, classify her as *Australopithecus afarensis*. She was vegetarian, eating grasses and leaves, as well as fruit, nuts, seeds, and tubers.[119]

### Homo Sapiens Harvested Wild Grains

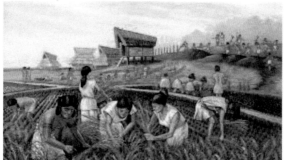

*Homo sapiens* have been harvesting wild grain, processing, and consuming it for at least half of its existence

Stone tools recently found in East Africa, the cradle of humanity, showed that people were processing sorghum 100,000 years ago. In Ngalue, a cave in Mozambique, researchers discovered an assortment of seventy stone tools in a layer of sediment deposited on the cave floor 42,000 to 105,000 years ago. Although the tools cannot be dated precisely, those in the deepest strata appear to be at least 100,000 years old. About 80% of the tools, including scrapers, grinders, points, flakes, and drills, had ample starchy residue, archaeologists told *Science*.[120] Eighty-nine percent of the starches came from sorghum, a cereal grain that still constitutes a main staple in many parts of Africa. The rest came from the African wine palm, the false banana, pigeon peas, wild oranges, and the African potato. The evidence suggests that people living in Ngalue routinely brought starchy plants, especially sorghum, to their cave where it was made into porridge and baked in the form of flat bread.

### Prehistoric European Bakeries

In multiple European sites, including present-day Moravia, Italy, and Russia, evidence has surfaced of ancient grain harvesting, cooking, and processing dating to about 25,000 to 30,000 years ago, a Stone Age era renowned for its elegant Ice Age cave paintings. For example, mammoth hunters in Dolni Vestonice, an Upper Paleolithic site in Moravia, had sickle blades and grinding stones. Researchers speculate that they harvested edible seeds of wild grasses, the common reed, bog bean, water nut, and arctic berries.[121] Remains of plant food preserved by a hearth at Dolni Vestonice II dating to from 27,000 to 24,000 years ago contained a seed, tissues from roots and tubers, possible acorn mush, and wood charcoal. In the Black Sea region, archaeologists unearthed thousands of small blades made of flint and hafted with bitumen into bone handles to harvest wild grasses and cane. As Dr Revedin of the Italian Institute of Prehistory and Early History in Florence concluded: "The discovery of grain and plant residues on grinding stones at the three sites suggests plant-based food processing, and possibly flour production, was common and widespread across Europe at least 30,000 years ago."[122]

## Food and Agriculture

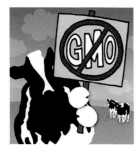

The introduction of genetically engineered foods in the 1990s fundamentally altered the human food supply. The Sacramento Valley in northern California is the site of most of the organic brown rice production in the United States. In 2000, Monsanto announced plans to introduce GMO rice in the region, a step that would almost certainly have resulted in the contamination of organic rice and the main staple in the macrobiotic community. Macrobiotic teachers Alex Jack, Edward Esko, Bettina Zumdick, and their associates formed Amberwaves, a grassroots network to educate the public about the potential dangers of genetically engineered crops. The campaign included a petition that garnered tens of thousands of signatures, concerts known as Amberfests, workshops and lectures,

The macrobiotic community mobilized to protect rice, wheat, and other key foods from genetic engineering

books and articles, and meetings with the California Rice Commission, FDA, EPA, and members of Congress. In the end, Monsanto was defeated, and GMO rice was never commercialized in the United States or elsewhere in the world. Amberwaves also helped prevented Monsanto from introducing GMO wheat.[123]

### ⚕ GMO Foods Imperil Natural Evolution

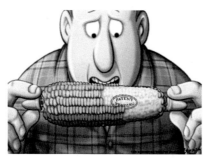

In a review of more than 100 scientific and medical studies on genetically engineered seeds, crops, and foods, an Amberwaves researcher concluded that GMOs pose a serious threat to continued natural biological and spiritual evolution. "Even before genetic engineering was developed, an estimated 97 percent of all native species of grains, beans, vegetables, and fruits in America disappeared in the 20th century, driven to extinction by monoculture, hybrid seeds, jet transportation, and modern economies of scale . . . It will take dramatic concerted action to protect freedom of choice, end the war on nature, and ensure the health of American and the planet as a whole."[124]

### ⵟ GMO Rice Harmful to Human Health

LibertyLink Rice, the first GMO rice developed in America, was grown experimentally in Texas in 2001. Amberwaves commissioned Joe Cummins, a Canadian geneticist who has written more than 200 research papers, to prepare a scientific report on LibertyLink Rice and its possible effects on human health and the environment. LL Rice is spliced with a gene that is resistant to glufosinate, an extremely toxic herbicide. In his study, Cummins reported that LibertyLink Rice would probably result in major adverse health effects to consumers and farmers, as well as reduced yields and the contamination of other plants.

"Glufosinate is a herbicide that kills almost everything green; it is used extensively with genetically engineered crops including corn, canola, and soybeans," he explained. "The herbicide resistant crops were approved by the Canadian and United States governments, even though there was clear evidence that the herbicide caused birth defects in experimental animals. The chemical acts by causing premature cell death in the immature brain by a process called apotosis. It also prevents development of glutamate channels in the brain, thus disrupting cellular communication. The birth defects observed in animals included brain defects leading to behavioral changes. Cleft lip and skeletal defects or kidney and urethra injury were observed in treated newborn. The herbicide also caused miscarriage and reduced conception in treated mothers. Exposure of male farm workers caused birth defects in their children."

As a result of a public campaign against GMO foods and the contamination of much of the nation's corn crop by an unapproved variety of modified corn, Aventis destroyed all 5 million pounds of LL Rice grown in Texas. Since then, there has been no commercialization of GMO rice.[125]

## Crime and Violence

Food affects mood as well as physical health. Macrobiotic food has figured prominently in several prison projects and helped reduce crime and violence.

### ⵟ Sugar Linked to Violent Behavior

Frank Kern, assistant director at Tidewater Detention Center in Chesapeake, Virginia, a state facility for juvenile offenders, initiated a double-blind dietary study. In 1979, Kern, a graduate of the Kushi Institute, arranged an experiment in which sugar was taken out of the meals and snacks of 24 inmates. Researchers found that the youngsters on the modified diet exhibited a 45 percent lower incidence of formal disciplinary actions and antisocial behavior than the control group. Follow-up studies showed that after limiting sugar there was an 82 percent reduction in assaults, 77 percent reduction in thefts, 65 percent reduction in horseplay, and 55 percent reduction in not obeying orders. The researchers also found that "the people most likely to show improvement were those who had committed violent acts on the outside." The findings appeared in *International Journal of Biosocial Research.*[126]

## Portuguese Prisoners Go Macrobiotic

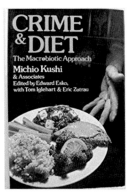

CRIME & DIET
The Macrobiotic Approach
Michio Kushi
& Associates
Edited by Edward Esko,
with Tom Iglehart & Eric Zutrau

In prison, many inmates started macrobiotics and became peaceful and went on to productive lives

In 1979 several inmates at the Central Prison in Linho, a maximum security facility, outside of Lisbon, Portugal, began eating a macrobiotic diet and attending lectures on Oriental philosophy and medicine. Soon 30 prisoners had become macrobiotic, including Toze Areal, the leader of a bank robber gang, and prison officials allowed them to use a large kitchen where they cooked and ate together several times a week. As a result of attitude and behavioral changes, most of the prisoners attending classes received commutations and were released early. "[T]here is a great difference in them, especially in those who have left the prison," Senhor Alfonso, a prison administrator, noted, commenting on the macrobiotic group. "It is not easy to describe—for one thing I can say that now they take more initiative. Actually, there is no problem here with anyone who is macrobiotic; this way of life enjoys a very good reputation. I believe the food and the outside stimulus both helped. The food can change people." Areal went on to study at the Kushi Institute, marry and have a large family, and start a company that made tofu and tempeh.[127]

## GMOs Linked to Sexual Decline and School Violence

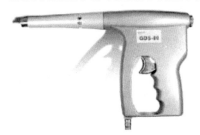

In a review of scientific and medical studies on GMOs, Alex Jack concluded that genetic engineering is contributing to abnormal sexual development, increased problems with conception, diminished sexual desire and perfor-

There may be a link between the outbreak of school shootings and consumption of GMO food strains created by the gene gun

mance, sex reversals and altered sex ratios, sterility, and other reproductive ills. He also examined the energetic effects of eating food produced from strains of GMO seeds developed with a gene gun—a pisto shooting modiified.22 and .45 bullets coated with genetic material into the plant—and correlated the introduction of GMO foods with the increase of violence in society, especially among children and the dramatic increase in shootings and other violent incidents in schools.[128]

## Peace and Social Justice

The Far Eastern word for peace is *wa* and is made up of two characters, or ideograms, for "grain" and "mouth." By eating a balanced whole grain diet, humans become calm and peaceful, see clearly, and exercise sound judgment. The Prophet Isaiah's dictum to turn swords into plowshares points at the same truth: peace comes from cultivating grains and eating in a plant-based way. Macrobiotic initiatives in the Middle East, South America, and other regions have helped reduce religious, ethnic, and class tensions and restore balance and harmony.

### Macrobiotic Food Unifies Warring Religions in Lebanon

Susana Sarué left the Sorbonne in Paris where she was completing her doctorate in nutrition to travel to the Middle East and used macrobiotic food and principles to help restore peace between warring Christians and Moslems in Beirut, as well as Palestinian refugees caught in the fighting, and Israeli soldiers and officials. She learned that there used to be a whole grain bread in Lebanon called Wise Bread because it gave wisdom, or nourishment, but for many years the bread had been

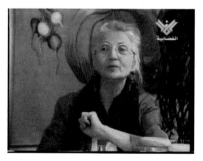

Miriam Nour, known as the Oprah of the Middle East, spreads macrobiotics through her daily TV show

made entirely with white flour. This flat bread composed about two-thirds of the daily diet. With donations, she and other macrobiotic practitioners opened a small bakery and brought the bread to the homes of many families who had a lot of children and who didn't have any work.

Gradually people learned how to make the bread themselves. Later, a natural foods cooperative was set up and made grains, beans, miso, soy sauce, and other healthy foods available. In East Beirut,

Miriam Nour, a prominent journalist, began to work in the villages and eventually became the leading macrobiotic teacher after Susana returned home. "Other countries—America, France—send us donations: canned food, sugar, white flour, margarine," Nour observed. "And they send us free medication. It's a vicious circle—the food is eaten, the people get sick, they go to hospitals, they take the medications. The food is eaten, the people become more aggressive, angry, and warlike. And the people who send this junk food and medication, the synthetic clothing, also send the bombs. It is also they who say they want to make peace. But the war itself wants to fight because there is war in our hearts and minds." Nour went on to host the leading TV talk show in the Middle East and introduced macrobiotics to millions of people, including the leaders of many Islamic countries.[129]

### Sugarcane Workers Gain Reforms after Dietary Change

In Virareka, a small village in Colombia, a sugarcane plantation had displaced local farms and fields. Over the years, large amounts of chemicals were applied to the cane, which came to displace all other crops. Deserts replaced green fields of grains and vegetables. Almost all the food eaten locally was brought in and consisted mainly of white flour, sugar, dairy food, meat, and other highly processed foods. Nutritionist Susana Sarué, a native of Latin America, returned to Colombia in the 1970s and developed a whole range of foods made from natural ingredients. She introduced a variety of cutlets, burgers, and other "meats" with a soya base, offered the people soy milk instead of dairy, and made an ice cream from sorghum and soya. The children's condition began to improve quickly. They became more alert and intelligent in school and less famished. They no longer had large stomachs. They also became more active. A health food bar was opened and managed by the local people. One day, the men of the village went on strike, and the bosses at the sugar plantation refused their demands, reasoning that they would starve after the third day and return to work. But the strikers, subsisting on local grains and beans and soy products, continued for two weeks, and the company was forced to give in and raise their wages.[130]

### Teaching Macrobiotics in War-Torn Syria

As the war in Syria spread, America and Russia initiated air strikes, and millions of refugees fled the country, Baydaa Laylaa, an elementary schoolteacher from Latakia, was busy giving macrobiotic cooking classes. Because of the war, the price of meat increased and people reduced

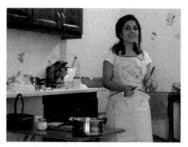

**Baydda Laylaa gave cooking classes in Syria.**

their consumption. Because of sanctions, pharmacies are offering whole foods and herbal remedies instead of drugs. Sanctions have also reduced the availability of macrobiotic specialty foods. Fighting has disrupted organic farming, so vegetables have been in short supply. After marrying Hussain Muhammad, another graduate of the Kushi Institute in America, Baydaa moved to Kuwait with her husband, but the couple still returns to Syria periodically to teach and give health consultations. In the future, they would like to start an organic farm. "There is no organic farming now," she noted. "Organic produce is imported, but it is expensive and the Ki energy is depleted. We also want to start a macrobiotic kitchen and introduce a healthier way of eating to children, parents, and the general public."[131]

### Trauma Teams Aid Children in Asia

Through Fortunate Blessings Foundation, Bill and Joan Spear, macrobiotic teachers in Litchfield, Connecticut, began an international relief program in 2004 to assist children who had been traumatized from natural disasters, war, torture, and other misfortune. After the initial emergency phase of a disaster, Second Response Trauma Teams, staffed by mental health professionals, travel to the impacted area to offer emotional support. During PLAYshops, participants directly engage in an experiential session on methodologies that employ body or somatic exercises to release repressed emotions. In recent years, trauma teams have assisted children in Sri Lanka and Indonesia following the great tsunami, as well as victims of the Nepalese earthquake and the nuclear accident at Fukushima in Japan.[132]

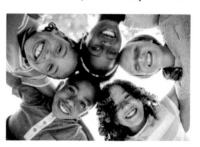

**Second Response aids children following natural disasters, war, and nuclear accidents**

# Planetary Health

The macrobiotic way of eating is beneficial for the planet as well as personal and social health. It helps protect the soil, air, water, and other natural resources from artificial fertilizers, pesticides, and other chemicals. It respects the diversity of species and contributes to the flourishing of bees, butterflies, and other pollinators. It reduces greenhouse gases in the atmosphere and mitigates climate change. Conversely, the modern way of farming and eating is a main cause of global warming, climate change, and other environmental destruction.

## Nutrient Decline

### ⚕ Nutrients in Produce Decline 25 to 50 Percent

In an analysis of the latest U.S. Department of Agriculture food composition tables, macrobiotic researcher Alex Jack reported a sharp decline in minerals, vitamins, and other nutrients in many chemically grown common foods between 1997 and 1975 when the last comprehensive survey was published. A random sampling of twelve garden vegetables found that calcium levels declined on average 26.5 percent, vitamin A dropped 21.4 percent, and vitamin C fell 29.9 percent. Whole grains and beans also showed sharp fluctuations. The amount of calcium and iron in millet fell 60 percent and 55.7 percent, and thiamin and riboflavin declined 42.3 percent and 23.7 percent, but niacin rose 105.2 percent. Brown rice also showed mixed results, with slight decreases in calcium and riboflavin, and mild increases in iron, thiamine, and niacin. Overall, green leafy vegetables appeared to have lost the most nutrients, while root vegetables, beans, and grains lost the least. "Decline of the natural environment appears to be the major reason for the widespread loss of nutrients. . . . This suggests a steady deterioration in soil, air, and water quality, as well as reduced seed vitality, that is depleting minerals and other inorganic components of food," the study concluded. Following an Open Letter to the U.S. Secretary of Agriculture by the editors of *Organic Gardening*, the USDA verified the accuracy of the study, and it was confirmed by other researchers.[133]

## Global Warming

### ⚕ Modern Diet Main Cause of Global Warming

Livestock's Long Shadow, the landmark report of the United Nation's Food and Agricultural Organization (FAO) concluded, the modern food pattern is the key to preventing warming, climate change, and othr environmental destruction. The study found that the cattle and other livestock industries are the single biggest contributor to global warming,

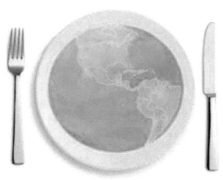

According to the United Nations, the modern food and agricultural system is the biggest contributor to climate change

"responsible for 18% of greenhouse gas emissions measured by CO2 equivalent. This is a higher share than transport," or 40 percent more than all the cars, trucks, buses, trains, and planes combined. The meat industry is "one of the . . . most significant contributors to the most serious environmental problems, at every scale from local to global," including "problems of land degradation, climate change and air pollution, water shortage and water pollution, and loss of biodiversity." Global meat and milk consumption is expected to double by 2050, further accelerating environmental destruction and global warming.[134]

### ☥ Dietary Change Saves More CO2 Than Buying a Prius

A 2006 study by Gidon Eishel and Pamela Martin at the University of Chicago found that a vegetarian diet is more energy efficient than one containing meat. The authors gathered data from many sources, examining the amount of fossil fuel energy required to sustain several different diets. The vegetarian diet turned out to be the most energy efficient, followed by a poultry-based diet and the standard American diet high in red meat. The authors compared a Toyota Prius, which uses about a quarter as much as fuel as a Chevrolet Suburban SUV, to a plant-based diet, which uses roughly one-fourth as much energy as a diet rich in red meat. Changing from a diet rich in red meat to a plant-based diet cuts greenhouse gas emissions as much as shifting from a Suburban SUV to a Prius.[135]

### ☥ Global Warming Alters Food Composition

Global warming is dramatically altering the nutritional value of foods worldwide. As a result of rising CO2 levels in the atmosphere, protein and nitrogen concentrations are down up to 25 percent in wheat, rice, and other major staples, mineral and trace element content have fallen 8 percent on average in 130 common crops, and carbohydrate has soared from 10 to 45 percent, according to the first ecological study of its kind. The dramatic increase in starch and sugar content may be the main cause of "hidden hunger" and the global obesity epidemic.

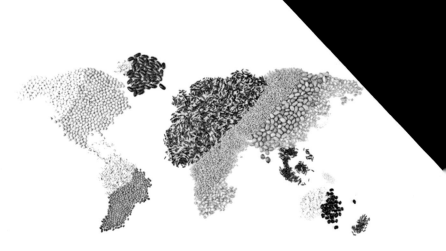

Elevated CO2 levels have reduced the overall concentration of 25 important minerals, including calcium, iron, potassium, and zinc, in plants by an average of 8 percent. The reduction in the nutritional value of crops could have profound impacts on human health. A mineral-deficient diet can cause malnutrition, even if a person consumes adequate calories. This pattern of eating is common in developing countries because most people eat a limited number of staples. Diets low in minerals, especially iron and zinc, lead to reduced growth in childhood, to reduced natural immunity and protection from infection, and higher rates of maternal and child deaths and sickness.

The study suggests that the altered nutrient profiles are contributing to the rise in obesity, as people eat too many high starch foods to begin with, and now as the earth warms these foods are increasing their proportion of simple sugars. Consumers also eat more to compensate for the lower mineral content in other foods. "The new evidence supports an emerging view that while obesity is quantified as an imbalance between energy inputs and expenditures, it could also be a form of malnutrition, where increased carbohydrate:protein and excessive carbohydrate consumption could be possible targets," observed Irakli Loladze, a mathematical biologist and quantitative ecologist, at the University of Maryland University College.

The study acknowledges that mineral declines in crops may be a consequence of the Green Revolution that relied on increased amounts of pesticides and artificial fertilizers that depleted the soil and altered mineral content.[136]

## Electromagnetic Fields

The electronics and digital revolution has bathed the planet in artificial electromagnetic radiation from satellites, televisions, cell phones, computers, tablets, smart meters, and other devices known as the Internet of Things. The long-term effects on human health and the environment are unknown. However, short-

d cell phones to brain tumors and disruption of glucose
disrupt wildlife, including the navigation systems of bees,
llinators that are crucial to the world food supply.

### Disrupt Bees

tists reported that the electromagnetic radiation emitted
es and base stations can interfere with the bees' navigation systems, rendering them unable to find their way back to their
hives. In an experiment conducted by researchers at Landau University,
bees refused to return to a hive when a mobile phone was placed near-
by. Although not conclusive, the experiment offers one possible explanation for the mysterious worldwide decline in the bee population known
as Colony Collapse Disorder (CCD). Other factors, including pesticides,
the varroa mite, viruses, genetically modified crops, and unusually cold
winters, are also believed to contribute to the decline.[137]

### Cell Phones Linked to Brain Tumors

In the most conclusive study to date linking non-ionizing cell phone radiation to brain cancer, research conducted by the National Toxicology
Program (NTP) reported in 2016 that rats exposed to RF (radio frequency) radiation had higher rates of glioma (a type of brain tumor), as well
as malignant schwannoma (a very rare heart tumor) than unexposed
rates. Radiation exposure showed a direct dose-response relationship.
Otis W. Brawley, M.D., chief medical officer for the American Cancer Society, stated: "The NTP report linking radiofrequency radiation (RFR) to
two types of cancer marks a paradigm shift in our understanding of radiation and cancer risk."[138]

## Energy and Transmutation

In 1959 French scientist Louis Kervran started publishing his discoveries in the
field of biological transmutation—the synthesis of necessary, but unavailable,
chemical elements out of simpler, available ones. He showed that in living biological systems sodium could change into potassium, manganese could be obtained
from iron, silica from calcium, and phosphorus from sulfur. Macrobiotic educator
George Ohsawa affirmed these findings, which flew in the face of conventional
physics and chemistry. He had long taught that everything in the universe is sub-
ject to the law of change and that transmutation of elements at ordinary temperatures and pressures was possible. Critics dismissed this view as alchemy, con-
tending that such transmutations could only occur under stellar or nuclear conditions. Michio Kushi assisted Ohsawa in several experiments verifying the process
and went on to herald the discovery as the catalyst for a new industrial revolution. He predicted that it would eventually replace mining and its toll on human life and environmental destruction and make valuable resources commonly
available for the betterment of society and a sustainable future.

### ♆ Saharan Workers Transmute Sodium to Potassium in Body

In 1959 French scientist Louis Kervran started publishing his discoveries in the field of biological transmutation —the synthesis of necessary but unavailable chemical elements out of simpler, available ones. His interest in this field began when he studied workers in the Sahara desert, who excreted more sodium than they consumed. Tests showed a comparable amount of potassium was being taken. Kervran showed potassium was capable of being transmuted into sodium in the body. Developing the theories of George Ohsawa that elements can be

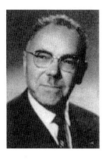

transmuted into one another peacefully without smashing the atom, Kervran went on to find that iron could be made from manganese, silica from calcium, and phosphorus from sulfur. Kervran's experiments have wide industrial, scientific, and social applications. For example, biological transmutations could be applied to rendering harmless nuclear wastes, toxic spills, and other chronic environmental hazards.[139]

**Louis Kervran, pioneer investigator of biological transmutation**

### ♆ Changing Carbon into Iron

Seeking to replicate Kervran's sodium to potassium experiment in the laboratory, George Ohsawa conducted a tabletop test in Tokyo in the early 1960s. Inserting positively and negatively charged electrodes into a vacuum tube, 2.3 mg of sodium combined with 1.6 mg of oxygen allowed to enter the tube and formed 3.9 mg of potassium. In another experiment, Ohsawa used a graphite crucible to transmute carbon into iron. He subsequently conducted other experiments until his death in 1966.[140]

### ♆ Pentagon Verifies Transmutation

U.S. military scientists tested the theory of biological transmutations and in 1978 verified the transmutation of matter from cell to cell and atom to atom. Surveying the works of Kervran and Ohsawa, researchers concluded "granted the existence of such transmutations (Na to Mg, K to Ca, and Mn to Fe), then a net surplus of energy was also produced. A proposed mechanism was described in which Mg adenosine triphosphate, located in the mitochondrion of the cell, played a double role as an energy producer. . . . The relatively available huge supplies of the elements which have been reported to have been transmuted and the probable large accompanying energy surplus indicate a new source of energy may be in the offing—one whose supply would be unlimited."[141]

### ⚕ 20 Key Industrial Elements Created

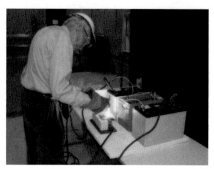

**Woody Johnson conducting carbon arc studies for Quantum Rabbit**

Quantum Rabbit LLC, a small macrobiotic company based in Massachusetts, transmuted small amounts of elements in a series of experiments between 2005 and 2016. In carbon-arc studies based on the Ohsawa/Kushi model, the QR team, consisting of Edward Esko, Alex Jack, and Woodward Johnson, produced from pure graphite (carbon) iron, magne sium, aluminum, silicon, scandium, titanium, cobalt, and nickel. Neodymium magnets showed the presence of magnetic activity, and an independent laboratory confirmed the presence of the metals in treated samples. A series of vacuum tube studies on noble gases fused helium plasma with oxygen to produce trace amounts of argon. In alkali metal vapor tests under vacuum, the QR team was able to produce potassium, copper, tin, germanium, and other elements. The QR researchers were able to produce potassium, palladium, strontium, silver, and gold. Results of more than a dozen studies were published in *Infinite Energy*, a journal dedicated to clean new energy sources.[142]

## Light Pollution

### ⚕ Dark Skies Vanishing

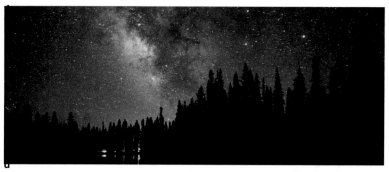

**80% of the world lives under light-polluted skies and can't see the Milky Way**

A new atlas of artificial night sky brightness shows that more than 80% of the world population and more than 99% of Americans, Europeans, and Japanese live under light-polluted skies.[143] Researchers report that the Milky Way is not visible to 80% of Americans and 60% of Europeans. This also includes Iraq, Syria, and other parts of the Middle East, where warfare has artificially lit up the sky.

Principal sources of light pollution are residential lights, streetlights, highway lights, motor vehicle headlights, sport stadium lights, electronic advertising billboards, shopping mall lights, park lights, airport lights, and offshore oil platforms.

The artificial light around cities and extending into many rural areas has interfered with the migration of nocturnal birds because they cannot follow the moon and stars. Light pollution also disorients bats, moths, and other animals that come out at night, and millions are killed each year by flying into streetlights. The metabolism of turtles, snakes, salamanders, and frogs has also been altered, as well as many plants.

Light pollution also affects humans, disrupting sleep, causing headaches, affecting sensory nerves, and contributing to depression. Alteration of circadian rhythms is further believed to increase the risk of obesity and diabetes. Some medical researchers suggest that artificial light, especially the blue component in white light at night, is carcinogenic.

From a macrobiotic perspective, the Milky Way and other stars shape and influence biological and spiritual evolution. As an article in *Amberwaves* noted: "They constantly charge our mid and forebrains, eyes, chakras, meridians, and other systems, organs, and functions, especially if we eat whole cereal grains that have awns or small antennae that receive and concentrate this cosmic energy and vibration. This current of incoming spiral energy orients us to beauty, truth, peace, justice, freedom, and other universal ideals. With the eclipse of night, the consciousness of modern society is rapidly dimming. . . .By respecting the natural rhythms and cycles of nature, including day and night, humanity can pass safely through this time. We can recover the compass of yin and yang, apply it to problems of society, and create a naturally bright new era."[144]

## The Coming Era

"The macrobiotic revolution is the most peaceful and effective way to restore the earth," as Michio Kushi observed. "Through it we are able to save ourselves and our families and friends from the vast current of degeneration sweeping the globe. We are even able to turn the general trend of modern civilization in a healthier, constructive direction. And, ultimately, we are able to enter the gateway of the new world, the Era of Humanity, with health and peace, justice and freedom, leading toward the unlimited happiness of all humanity for endless generations to come."[145]

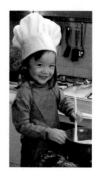

**Despite all the challenges, the macrobiotic community sees a bright, happy future for the planet and future generations**

# Daily Menu and Recipes

The following recipes are for a typical macrobiotic meal, including breakfast, lunch, midafternoon snack, and dinner. Amounts are for 3–4 people.

## BREAKFAST

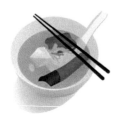

### Miso Soup

2-inch piece of dried wakame sea vegetable
1 cup onions, sliced thinly
1 quart water
barley miso

Soak the wakame (about ¼-½-inch piece per person) for 5 minutes and cut into small pieces. Add the wakame to fresh, cold water and bring to a boil. Meanwhile, cut onions into small pieces. Add the vegetables to the boiling broth and boil all together for 3-5 minutes until the vegetables are soft and edible. Reduce flame to low. Dilute miso (½ to 1 level teaspoon per cup of broth) in a little water, add to soup, and simmer for 3-4 minutes on a low flame. Once the miso is added, don't boil the soup. Just let it simmer. Garnish with finely chopped scallions or parsley before serving.

- Be sure to simmer the soup for 3-4 minutes *after* miso paste is added to the broth. This is a very simple soup to make, but not letting the miso cook properly will reduce its effects
- For variety or a gluten-free miso, use brown rice miso or all soybean (hatcho). As a rule, misos for daily soup should be aged a minimum of 2 years. Misos may also be combined for a unique taste and flavor. Lighter red, yellow, and white misos make great dressings and sauces
- Vary the vegetables daily. Nice combinations include onions and tofu; onions and sweet autumn or winter squash; cabbage and carrots; and daikon and daikon greens
- Include leafy greens often in miso soup, including kale, collards, watercress, etc. Add them toward the end of cooking since they don't need to cook as long

- A small volume of shiitake mushrooms (soaked and finely chopped beforehand) may be added and cooked with the other vegetables from time to time
- For the most beneficial effect, miso soup should be cooked fresh each time and not stored overnight

## Millet and Squash Porridge

This recipe makes a delight, sweet morning porridge the whole family will enjoy.

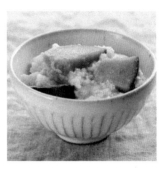

1 cup millet
½ cup butternut or other squash, sliced into small chunks
pinch of sea salt
3 to 4 cups water

Wash millet in cold water and place in a saucepan. Add fresh cooking water and seasoning. Bring to a boil, lower flame, and add cut up squash. Cover and let simmer for about 20-25 minutes. Garnish with chopped scallions, parsley, gomashio (sesame seed salt), or other condiment. This makes a sweet, delicious morning porridge and is also very strengthening.

## Steamed Greens

Kale, collards, watercress, mustard greens, dandelion greens, carrot tops, Chinese cabbage, or other greens

Wash and slice any of the above vegetables. Place the vegetables in a small amount of water, about ½ inch, or in a stainless steel steamer over 1 inch of boiling water. Cover and steam or boil for 2-3 minutes, depending on the texture of the vegetables. Transfer quickly to a serving dish to prevent overcooking.

- The vegetables should be a bright green color and crispy
- Wait until the water is fully boiling before you put in the vegetables
- You may lightly sprinkle shoyu over the greens at the end of the cooking
- You may serve plain or occasionally add a few drops of brown rice or umeboshi vinegar
- When boiling, do not cover the pot with a lid or the greens will lose their bright green color

## Bancha Twig Tea

Bancha twig tea is served as the principal beverage in most macrobiotic households. It is usually available dry-roasted and is often marketed as *kukicha*. It consists of the twigs or stems of the tea plant. Green tea is made from the leaves of the tea plant, while black tea is made from leaves that have been dyed. The leaves are high in caffeine, while the twigs and stems are virtually caffeine-free. To make tea, add a tablespoon of twigs to 1 quart of water and bring to a boil. Lower flame and simmer for several minutes. Place tea strainer in cup and pour out tea. Twigs in strainer may be returned to teapot and used several times, adding a few fresh twigs each time.

# LUNCH

## Udon Noodles in Broth with Tofu and Watercress

Udon or whole wheat noodles in broth with tofu and veggies make a tasty lunch.

1 package udon noodles
2 ounces tofu, cut in small cubes
½ cup watercress
2 dried shiitake mushrooms
1 piece of kombu, 2-3 inches long
4 cups water
2-3 tablespoons shoyu

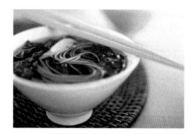

Add noodles to a pan of rapidly boiling water. No salt is needed. After about 10 minutes, check to see if they are done by breaking the end of one noodle. If the inside and outside are the same color, noodles are ready. If the inside is white or lighter, cook some more until done. Remove noodles from pot, strain, and rinse with cold water to stop from cooking and prevent clumping.

Steam tofu and watercress separately for 5 minutes each. To retain the bright green color, don't overcook. Place on top of noodles when done.

For the broth, place kombu in a saucepan, add 4 cups of water and mushrooms that have been soaked, stems removed, and sliced. Bring to a boil, reduce flame, and simmer for 3-5 minutes. Remove kombu and shiitake. Add shoyu to taste and simmer for another 3-5 minutes. Serve noodles with hot broth and garnish with scallions, chives, or toasted nori.

• Grated ginger may be added to the broth
• For variety use other Eastern style noodles such as soba and somen. Western style whole grain noodles and pasta may also be used, including spaghetti, shells, spirals, elbows, flat noodles, and lasagna. Add a pinch of salt in cooking

## Garden Salad with Poppy Seed Vinaigrette

A variety of fresh, uncooked vegetables may be used in this preparation. In addition to lettuce, these include cabbage, grated carrots, radishes, cucumbers, celery, and arugula.

• Variation: Rice, bulghur, couscous, or other grain placed on a bed of lettuce with some of these vegetables makes a tasty meal in the spring or summer.

*Poppy Seed Vinaigrette*

Makes 1 1/4 cups

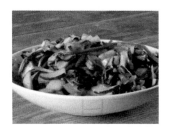

1/4 cup lemon juice
zest from 1 lemon
1 teaspoon Dijon mustard
2 tablespoons rice syrup
1/4 cup chopped onions
2 teaspoons shoyu
5 tablespoons olive oil
pinch of sea salt to taste
3 tablespoons poppy seeds, lightly toasted

Place all the ingredients except poppy seeds in a blender. Blend until the texture is smooth. Place the mixture in a mixing bowl. Add poppy seeds, and mix well with a whisk. Adjust consistency and flavor if necessary. Store leftover vinaigrette in a jar and keep in refrigerator for 3–4 days.

## Roasted Barley Tea

Roasted barley tea is very relaxing, especially in the spring or summer. This tea can also be purchased pre-roasted.

Makes 3 cups
½ cup uncooked barley
1½ tablespoons roasted rice
3/4 cup water

Dry-roast uncooked barley in a skillet. Stir and shake pan occasionally to prevent burning. Add 1½ to 2 tablespoons of roasted rice to 1 quart of water. Bring to a boil, reduce flame, and simmer for 10-15 minutes.

# MID-AFTERNOON SNACK

## Pan-Fried Mochi
8 ounces of mocha cut into 2-inch squares

Mochi is pounded sweet rice that is traditionally eaten as a festive dish or for special occasions. It can be made at home by pounding cooked sweet rice with a heavy wooden pestle in a wooden bowl. Pound until grains are crushed and become very sticky. Wet pestle occasionally to prevent rice from sticking to it. Form rice into small balls or cakes or spread on a baking sheet that has been oiled and dusted with flour and let dry. Mochi is also now available ready made in the natural foods store.

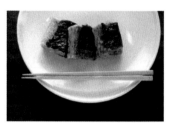

Cut mochi into small squares and place on a preheated skillet. No oil is necessary. Cover and cook over a low to medium flame for a few minutes until the mochi expands and puffs up. Check frequently or it will over expand and burst. Turn over and cook the other side. Eat plain or serve with a little barley malt for a sweet taste; a few drops of shoyu for a salty taste; or wrap in toasted nori.

## Fresh Carrot Juice
Carrot juice is a delightful beverage. If you use a juicer, let the electrical energy come down about 10 minutes before drinking.

# DINNER

## Brown Rice with Barley
2 cups brown rice
1/2 cup of barley
4 1/2 to 5 cups of water
2 pinches of sea salt

Wash the grains and place in a saucepan. When the water is warm, add the sea salt, put on the cover, and bring to a boil. Reduce flame and simmer for about 50 minutes. Let set for 5 minutes and gently remove from the pot.

• Other grains such as whole wheat berries, whole oats, millet, rye, and fresh corn kernels may be cooked in this way.

## Lentil Stew
1 cup lentil beans (sorted and washed)

1 small onion, diced
1 carrot or 1/2 cup winter squash, diced
2-inch square piece of kombu
2 cups water

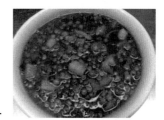

Dice the carrots and onions or squash. Layer kombu on the bottom of a pot and place lentils on top. Add water. Bring the contents to a boil without a lid, reduce the flame, and cook for about 30 minutes without a lid. Discard any foam that may rise to the surface. Add water was water evaporate covering the beans. Cover the pot and simmer on a low flame. Cook with low flame for approximately 40 minutes until beans become soft. Place vegetables on top of beans. Cover and continue to cook everything become soft. Flavor with a little shoyu or miso. Continue to simmer another five minutes. Transfer to a serving dish. Garnish with chopped parsley.

## Arame with Onions
1 ounce dried arame sea vegetable
1 tablespoon sesame oil
1 medium onion, sliced

Wash and drain arame. Brush a skillet with light or dark sesame oil and heat it. Add the onions and sauté for 2-3 minutes. (Water-sauté if oil is to be avoided.) Place the arame on top of the onions and add enough water to just cover the onions. Bring to a boil, turn the heat down to low, and add a small amount of shoyu. Cover and simmer for about 20-25 minutes. Add shoyu to taste, but dish should not be overly salty. Simmer for another 5-10 minutes, mix, and stir until the liquid has evaporated.

• Carrot, dried daikon, rutabaga, sweet corn, or other vegetables may also be added.

### Shoyu Pickles
Mix equal parts spring water and shoyu in a bowl or glass jar. Slice vegetables such as turnips or rutabaga and place in this liquid. Soak for 4 to 8 hours and serve.

• Pickles aid in digestion of grains and vegetables
• Sauerkraut may also be used

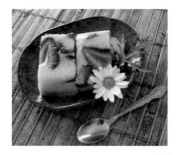

## Strawberry Kanten

1 cup strawberries, freshly sliced
2/3 cup apple juice per person

1/3 cup water per person
1/4 cup amasake (optional)
2 tablespoons agar agar flakes
1 teaspoon kuzu

Kanten is a delicious, mild gelatin. Made with agar-agar, a sea vegetable that is processed into flakes or powder, it is very light and refreshing.

Slice strawberries and set aside. Simmer liquid ingredients and agar flakes until the agar has dissolved. Dissolve kuzu in a few tablespoons of water and stir in mixture until it thickens. Pour liquid over the strawberries and serve.

• For variety, use peaches, apples, blueberries, cherries, cantaloupe, or other seasonal fruit, individually or in combination

**Bancha Twig Tea** (see p. 84)

# Home Remedies

### Carrot-Daikon Drink
This drink helps to dissolve hardened fat and oil deposits in the body and is a principal remedy to relieve heart disease, many tumors, and other disorders caused by too much saturated fat and oil intake. The daikon melts the hardened accumulations from within and discharges them through the urine.

Makes 2 cups
1/3 to ½ cup carrot, finely grated
½ cup daikon, finely grated
several drops of shyu
1/3 sheet nori
½ umeboshi plum

Finely grate the carrot and daikon and place in a saucepan. Add the nori and umeboshi plum. Add 1 to 1 ½ cups water and bring to a gentle boil. Simmer for about 3 minutes and add a few drops of shoyu toward the end. Eat and drink the vegetables and the broth.

### Ume-Sho-Kuzu
Ume-Sho Kuzu is a standard macrobiotic drink used to strengthen digestion, restore energy, reduce inflammation, and help the body discharge acidity.

Makes 1 cup

1 heaping teaspoon kuzu

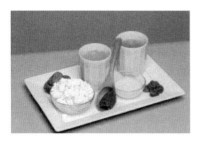

2–3 teaspoons cold water
½–1 teaspoon shoyu
1 cup bancha twig tea

**Ume-sho-kuzu aids digestion, prevents infection, and restores vitality**

Dissolve kuzu in cold water. Add one cup of cold water to the dissolved kuzu. Bring to a boil over a medium flame, stirring constantly to avoid lumping, until the liquid becomes translucent. Reduce the flame to low. Add the pulp of the umeboshi plum. Add several drops to 1 teaspoon of shoyu and stir gently. Simmer for 2–3 minutes and drink hot.

## Sweet Vegetable Drink

This drink was developed to help offset the effects of chicken, egg, and cheese consumption, leading to hypoglycemia, or chronic low blood sugar, a condition that affects about 75 or 80% of everyone in modern society. It is especially beneficial for softening the pancreas and helping to stabilize blood sugar levels. A small cup may be taken daily or every other day, especially in the mid- to late-afternoon. It will satisfy the desire for a sweet taste and help reduce cravings for simple sugars and other stronger sweets.

Use equal amounts of 4 sweet vegetables, finely chopped (onions, carrots, cabbage, and sweet winter squash). Boil 3 to 4 times the amount of water, add chopped vegetables, and allow to boil uncovered for 2 to 3 minutes. Reduce the flame to low, cover, and let simmer for 20 minutes. Strain the vegetables from the broth. (You may occasionally use them later in soups and stews.) Drink the broth, either hot or at room temperature.

- No seasoning is used in this recipe
- Sweet vegetable drink may be kept in the refrigerator for up to 2 days, but should be warmed again or allowed to return to room temperature before drinking

# Guidelines for Use of Supplements

Our daily diet is the foundation for our physical, mental, emotional, and spiritual health, as well as the means to maintain and supply the vital energy for social activity. If we properly manage our daily diet and harmonize with the environment, there is generally no need to take specific supplements. However, some persons may require supplements for a limited time:

- When a person is currently in a transition period from unhealthful eating habits to a well-balanced macrobiotic diet
- When a person is not eating a well-balanced macrobiotic diet but is only partially doing so
- When a person who has developed a serious illness that may require supplemental, convention, or alternative approaches until she or he establishes a

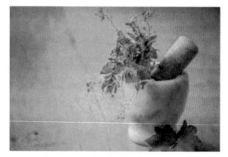

reasonably healthy condition and begins to practice a macrobiotic way of life
- When a person does not have access to high quality natural and organic foods because they are in a boarding school, the military, nursing home, prison, etc.

**Supplements include herbs, minerals and extracts.**

- When the natural or organic food supply has declined appreciably in Ki energy or nutrients or is contaminated by GMOs, heavy metals, or other toxins

The preferred quality of supplements is as follows beginning with the highest quality:

1. Supplements prepared at home using natural, preferably organic, whole food ingredients, including such common macrobiotic home remedies as Ume-Sho-Kuzu Tea, Carrot-Daikon Drink, Lotus Tea, and many others
2. Segments or extracts of natural plant-quality food, including grains, beans, vegetables, sea vegetables, roots, tubers, fruits, seeds, and nuts, that people can make themselves or purchase if available. Natural food processing methods include juicing, heating, pressing, drying, diluting, crushing, roasting, boiling, freezing, smoking, and other similar applications that do not involve the use of chemicals or synthetic products, chemical processing, high pressure, artificial aging, irradiation, or other extreme methods. Examples include vegetable and fruit juices, herbal teas, Chinese medicinal herbs (e.g. dong quai, ginseng), Native American herbs (e.g., slippery elm), spirulina,

blue green algae, green magma, and various homeopathic remedies (e.g., arnica)
3. Products that contain natural minerals, but are not coated, mixed, or treated with chemical or artificial substances. Preferably these minerals are from plant sources. Examples include "vegan" calcium, iron, magnesium, zinc, etc.
4. Products that contain 20% or less (by total weight of the product) meat, poultry, dairy, fish, seafood, or other animal-based substances and which contain no chemical additives or chemical processing. Examples include certain Chinese medicine, folk medicines, oyster shells, fossils, bones, skin, eggs
5. Products that contain natural plant, mineral, and animal substances as well as chemical substances or chemical processing, so long as their benefits outweigh their risks and harmful effects

Chemical, synthetic, and artificial supplements and medications should be avoided or reduced as much as possible. In some cases, for example, thyroid medication, patients are given a choice of a synthetic hormone or one made from pigs. The animal-quality is more natural than the synthetic and usually preferable.

If used at all, the above-mentioned supplements are best consumed on a temporary basis, while at the same time, the individual maintains a well-balanced macrobiotic dietary practice for optimal health benefits. It is not advisable to consume supplements for long periods of time, though certain medications (like the thyroid medication mentioned above) may need to be taken indefinitely. The period of use will differ for each case and fluctuate depending upon individual condition and needs. In the event a person requires taking supplements continuously for a prolonged period (over 6 months), then his or her daily practice of the macrobiotic way of eating should be thoroughly reviewed.

# Regional Guidelines
## 1. Temperate Regions

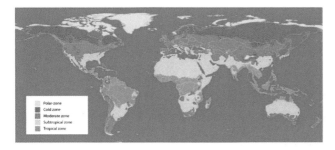

Including North America, Europe, Russia, China, East Asia, and Moderate Regions in Southern Africa, South America, Australia, and New Zealand

*Daily Food*
- Whole Cereal Grains: Brown rice, millet, whole wheat, barley, corn, and others (30-50%)
- Soup: Various (5-10%)
- Vegetables: Various (25-35%)
- Beans and Sea Vegetables: Various (5-10%)

*Plus supplemental foods and beverages:*
- Fish and seafood (optional)
- Local fruit, seeds, and nuts
- Natural Processed oils, seasonings, and condiments
- Natural Sweets
- Non-aromatic and nonstimulant beverages, and occasional aromatic and stimulant beverages

*Environmental Quality*
- Food to be organically grown as much as possible
- Water to be spring, well, or purified
- Fire to be from wood, charcoal, gas, solar, or other natural source

## 2. Central and South America
Including Mexico, Guatemala, Costa Rica, Panama, and the Caribbean Islands and Coastal Regions

*Daily Food*
- Whole Cereal Grains: Maize, amaranth, quinoa, brown rice, and other whole cereal grains and a portion consisting of tacos, chapatis, noodles and pasta, flat bread and others, as well as cassava, sweet potato, and potato (40-50%)
- Soup: Various (5-10%)
- Vegetables and Fruits: Various (25-35%)

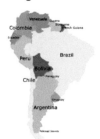

- Beans and Sea Vegetables including pinto, kidney, chickpeas, and water and river moss: Various (10-15%)

*Plus supplemental foods and beverages:*
- Fish and seafood, small game insects, or other animal food (optional)
- Local seeds and nuts, roots and tubers

94

- Natural Processed oils, seasonings, condiments and spices
- Natural Sweets
- Non-aromatic and nonstimulant beverages, and occasional aromatic and stimulant beverages

*Environmental Quality*
- Food to be organically grown as much as possible
- Water to be spring, well, or purified
- Fire to be from wood, charcoal, gas, solar, or other natural source

## 3. Middle East
Including Western Asia, the Arabian Peninsula, and Northern Africa
*Daily Food*

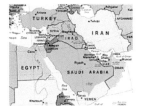

- Whole Cereal Grains: Barley, wheat, millet, long grain rice, couscous, bulghur, buckwheat, and others and grain products (40-50%)
- Animal Food: fish, lamb, camel's milk, poultry, etc. (optional) (10–20%)
- Soup: Various (5-10%)
- Vegetables and Fruits: Various (25-35%)
- Beans and Sea Vegetables including hummus, falafel, river and water moss: Various (5-10%)

*Plus supplemental foods and beverages:*
- Local seeds and nuts, roots and tubers
- Natural Processed oils, seasonings, condiments and spices
- Natural Sweets
- Non-aromatic and nonstimulant beverages, and occasional aromatic and stimulant beverages

*Environmental Quality*
- Food to be organically grown as much as possible
- Water to be spring, well, or purified
- Fire to be from wood, charcoal, gas, solar, or other natural source

## 4. Africa
including hot and equatorial regions of West, Central, East, and South Africa

*Daily Food*

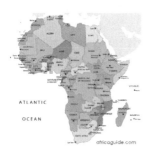

- Whole Cereal Grains and Tubers: millet, sorghum, teff, brown rice, corn, and others and a smaller portion of yams, sweet potato, and others(40-50%)
  - Soup: Various (5-10%)
  - Vegetables and Fruits: Various (25-35%)
  - Beans and Sea Vegetables including water, lake, and river moss: Various (5-10%)

*Plus supplemental foods and beverages:*
- Fish and seafood, small game, insects, or other animal food (optional)
- Local seeds and nuts, roots and tubers
- Natural Processed oils, seasonings, condiments and spices
- Natural Sweets
- Non-aromatic and nonstimulant beverages, and occasional aromatic and stimulant beverages

*Environmental Quality*
- Food to be organically grown as much as possible
- Water to be spring, well, or purified
- Fire to be from wood, charcoal, gas, solar, or other natural source

## 5. South Asia

Including India, Pakistan, Bangladesh, and Sri Lanka
*Daily Food*

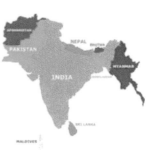

- Whole Cereal Grains: Basmati and long grain rice, millet, whole wheat, barley, and others and a
- smaller portion of chapatti, roti, dosa, and other flat breads (40-50%)
- Soup: Various (5-10%)
- Vegetables and Fruits: Various (25-35%)
- Beans and Sea Vegetables including dhal, chickpeas, and other legumes and river and water moss: Various (5-10%)

*Plus supplemental foods and beverages:*
- Fish and seafood (optional)
- Local seeds and nuts, roots and tubers
- Natural Processed oils, seasonings, condiments and spices
- Natural Sweets
- Non-aromatic and nonstimulant beverages, and occasional aromatic and stimulant beverages

*Environmental Quality*
- Food to be organically grown as much as possible
- Water to be spring, well, or purified
- Fire to be from wood, charcoal, gas, solar, or other natural source

## 6. Southeast Asia and the Pacific Islands

Including Thailand, Vietnam, Malaysia, Singapore, and Indonesia

*Daily Food*
- Whole Cereal Grains: Brown rice, millet, whole wheat, corn, and others and a smaller portion of noodles and pasta, dumplings, bread, and taro (40-50%)
- Soup: Various (5-10%)
- Vegetables and Fruits: Various (25-35%)
- Beans and Sea Vegetables including tofu, tempeh, and others (10-15%)

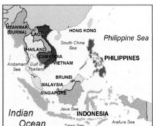

*Plus supplemental foods and beverages:*
- Fish and seafood, small game, insects, or other animal food (optional)
- Local seeds and nuts, roots and tubers
- Natural Processed oils, seasonings, condiments and spices
- Natural Sweets
- Non-aromatic and nonstimulant beverages, and occasional aromatic and stimulant beverages

*Environmental Quality*
- Food to be organically grown as much as possible
- Water to be spring, well, or purified
- Fire to be from wood, charcoal, gas, solar, or other natural source

# Trump Administration Jettisons U.S. Dietary Guidelines

## By Alex Jack

The 2020 U.S. Dietary Guidelines will be formulated by experts with ties to the beef, dairy, and sugar industries after the Trump Administration jettisoned the processed by which national nutritional recommendations have been issued for decades. The guidelines, revised and updated every five years, are used to administer school lunch, hospital, and food assistance programs around the country. Manufacturers use the guidelines to formulate products that the USDA and Department of Health and Human Services purchase for $100 billion annually.

All medical studies conducted before 2000 are off the table for consideration, including virtually all of the pioneer macrobiotic studies on blood pressure, cholesterol, and other heart values that formed the foundation of the original *Dietary Goals for the United States* report in 1977, the food pyramids in the 1980s and 90s, and the MyPlate recommendations of the 2000s. Similarly, the path-breaking studies on the superiority of mother's milk to infant formula have been dumped.

The list of preapproved topics the committee is allowed to discuss does not include the consumption of red and processed meat, the spread of highly processed foods, or the proper sodium levels for different populations or ages.

Nutritionists reacted in shock to the directives since these foods are widely held to be the underlying cause of atherosclerosis, heart disease, stroke, obesity, and type 2 diabetes. "The cutting-edge issues in dietary advice in 2019 are about eating less meat, avoidance of ultra-processed foods, and sustainable production and consumption," says Marion Nestle, author of *The Politics of Food* and a nutritionist at New York University. "Guidelines that avoid these issues will be years behind the times."

"The dietary guidelines are under assault from multiple directions," David Katz, director of Yale University's Yale Griffin Prevention Research Center, said. "This time around, veiled organizations representing the interests of beef, dairy, and Big Food are pretending to use science to argue against the actual science and to expunge key recommendations. Of course, sustainability should be included. Of course, we need to eat less meat."

In keeping with the Administration's denial of global warming, the new guidelines will ignore the relationship between food and climate change. Meanwhile, the United Nations, the World Resources Institute, the World Bank, and many other international institutions have called for dramatically lower amounts of beef and other animal food production to prevent the catastrophic impact of the climate crisis.

Danielle Beck, a spokesperson for the National Cattlemen's Beef Association, hailed the new approach, saying it preserves the integrity of the scientific process. "The guidelines were never intended to talk about sustainability; those questions are outside the scope of law," she said. "We're confident . . . it will acknowledge beef's role in a heart-healthy, balanced diet."

According to the Center for Science in the Public Interest, thirteen of the twenty experts on the 2020 dietary guidelines panel have ties to the food industry. Several were nominated by the National Cattlemen's Beef Association, the National Potato Council, and trade association of the snack food industry. Nine were recommended by the Academy of Nutrition and Dietitians, a pro-processed food group funded by McDonald's, Coca-Cola, and Mars.

The cozy relationship between giant food producers and the White House extends to other nutritional programs. The Food, Nutrition, and Consumer Services department is led by Maggie Lyons, a former lobbyist for the National Grocers Association, and Kailee Tkacz, a former lobbyist for the corn syrup and snack food industries. Tkacz received an ethical waiver to be employed by Donald McGahn, the former White House counsel who is a key figure in the Russian investigation.

# Glossary

**Agar-agar** A white gelatin processed from a sea vegetable used in cooking as a thickener in making aspics and kanten. Comes in flakes, powder, or bars and makes cool, refreshing dishes.

**Amazake** A cultured beverage or concentrate made from rice or other whole grains and *koji*. It makes delicious puddings, mousses, and other desserts.

**Arame** A wiry dark sea vegetable that turns dark brown when cooked.

**Azuki beans** Small red beans originally from the Far East but now grown in North America. They go especially well with squash and kombu. Also called aduki or adzuki.

**Bancha twig tea** Tea prepared from the twigs of the tea bush. High in calcium and other nutrients, it aids digestion and gives a calm, soothing energy. It contains no caffeine or dyes and is suitable for children and adults. Also known as *kukicha*.

**Barley** A traditional grain in the Mediterranean and Aegean world, the British Isles, Central Asia, and, most recently, North America. It is used in soup, stews, bread, and beer and gives light, upward energy.

**Barley malt** A thick dark-brown sweetener made from barley. It is used in desserts, to sweeten beans, and in medicinal preparations.

**Black soybeans** Shiny black soybeans are usually smaller and lower in fat than yellow soybeans. Also known as Japanese black beans.

**Blanched salad** A crisp, colorful salad made by lightly dipping different combinations of sliced vegetables into boiling water for thirty seconds to several minutes.

**Bok choy** A leafy green vegetable with thick white stems. Also known as pok choy.

**Brown rice** Unpolished rice that retains the germ, bran, and other outer layers of the whole grain. It contains an ideal balance of minerals, protein, and carbohydrates and gives strong, peaceful energy. It is available in several varieties, including short, medium, and long grain; sweet brown rice; basmati; and jasmine.

**Brown rice vinegar** A mild, delicate vinegar made from fermented brown rice or sweet brown rice. It is used in dressings, sauces, and medicinal drinks.

**Buckwheat** A cereal plant native to Siberia, Russia, and Eastern Europe. It is eaten in the form of kasha, whole groats, or soba noodles and gives strong, active energy.

**Burdock** A long, dark root vegetable that grows wild in many regions of the world. It is used in soups, stews, and *nishime-* and *kinpira*-style dishes and gives strengthening energy.

**Complex carbohydrates** The nutrients that provide the body with a continuous source of energy. Known chemically as polysaccharides, they are found in whole grains, beans, vegetables, and sea vegetables and form the main part of the macrobiotic diet.

**Couscous** A light steamed wheat product made from semolina, popular in the Middle East, North Africa, and France. It cooks up quickly and is used in light grain dishes, salads, and cakes.

**Daikon** A long white radish that is used in soups and veggie dishes or grated raw as a garnish. Its taste ranges from sweet to pungent and helps dissolve accumulations of fat and oil from the body. A shredded dried variety is used for special dishes and medicinal preparations.

**Dried Tofu** Tofu that has been dehydrated and frozen. Used in soups, stews, and veggie or sea veggie dishes. Less fatty than tofu.

**Dulse** A reddish-purple sea vegetable harvested in the North Atlantic Ocean. It is used in soups, salads, and side dishes and has a zesty flavor.

**Fermentation** The living activity of enzymes, bacteria, and yeast causes certain foods to change chemically and make them easier to digest and strengthens the intestinal flora. In the macrobiotic diet, fermented foods include miso, shoyu, *natto*, tempeh, amazake, brown rice or other vinegars, sourdough bread, sauerkraut, and pickles.

**Fiber** The indigestible cellulose part of whole foods, especially the bran of whole grains and the outer skin of beans, vegetables, and fruits. Fiber helps cleanse the intestines and protect against heart disease, cancer, and other diseases. Refined, processed, and peeled foods are low in fiber.

**Fu** A dried wheat-gluten product available in thin sheets or thick round cakes. It cooks up softly and adds protein and texture to soups, stews, and other dishes.

**Ginger** A spicy, pungent golden-colored root used in cooking as a seasoning, as a garnish, and for medicinal applications. It is primarily used fresh and grated with a small hand grater.

**Gluten** The protein component of wheat, barley, rye, and oats that gives elasticity to dough and a chewy texture when eaten. Gluten is used to make seitan and *fu*.

**Gomashio** Sesame salt made from roasted, ground sesame seeds and sea salt. The most popular condiment in macrobiotic cooking, it is sprinkled on brown rice and other whole grains.

**Grain coffee** A mild beverage made from roasted barley, acorns, chicory, or other plants and sometimes a natural sweetener. It is used like instant coffee and is free of caffeine and stimulating effects.

**Green nori flakes/Aonori** A sea vegetable condiment that is sprinkled on grains, vegetables, and salads. It is from a different variety of nori than the packaged variety available in sheets.

**Hijiki** A dark-brown sea vegetable that turns black when dried. It has a strong ocean taste and is rich in protein, calcium, and iron. It is imported from Japan or harvested off the Maine coast. Also known as *hiziki*.

**Kanten** A gelatin made from the agar-agar sea vegetable. It may include apples, berries, melons, or other fruits; amazake; azuki beans; and other foods. After cooking, it is usually chilled and served as a dessert or snack.

**Kasha** Buckwheat groats that are roasted and boiled.

**Ki** Natural electromagnetic energy from heaven and earth that vitalizes food, water, breath, and all living things. Known as chi in China, *prana* in India, and the Holy Spirit in the West.

**Kombu** A thick dark-green sea vegetable that grows in deep ocean water and is cooked with whole grains, beans, and vegetables. It is also used to make soup stocks, candy, and condiments.

**Kuzu** A fine white starch made from the root of the kuzu plant. It is used as a thickener in soups, sauces, desserts, and medicinal drinks. Also known as kudzu.

**Lotus** A water lily whose edible roots have a light-brown skin, long hollow chambers, and an off-white inside. The large white seeds are also eaten. Lotus is especially beneficial for the lungs and sinuses.

**Meridian** A stream of natural electromagnetic energy flowing through the human organism or other living things. Far Eastern medicine and philosophy, including dietetics, acupuncture, shiatsu, *do-in*, and the martial arts, are based on reestablishing the meridian flow, which can be impeded by improper diet and lifestyle.

**Millet** A small yellow grain native to China, India, Africa, and ancient Mesoamerica. It gives strong, balanced energy; has a mildly, sweet taste; and is especially good for the pancreas, stomach, spleen, and lymphatic functions. A glutinous variety is known as sweet millet or *kibi* millet.

**Miso** A nourishing, mildly-sweet-tasting paste or purée made from soybeans, sea salt, and usually fermented barley or brown rice. There are many varieties of miso that are used in making miso soup, seasoning other dishes, and preparing sauces and dressings. Miso contains enzymes and other compounds that facilitate digestion, strengthen the blood, and help protect against cancer, heart disease, and radiation sickness. It is used externally as a plaster.

**Mochi** A dumpling, cube, or cake made from steamed and pounded glutinous sweet brown rice. It is traditionally enjoyed on New Year's Day and is especially good for lactating mothers, as it promotes the production of breast milk.

**Natto** Soybeans that are cooked, mixed with beneficial enzymes, and allowed to ferment for twenty-four hours. High in protein and vitamin B12, natto is especially beneficial to digestion and strengthening the intestines.

**Nori** Thin sheets of a black or dark-purple dried sea vegetable that turns green when toasted over a flame. High in vitamins and minerals, it is used to make sushi, to wrap rice balls, and as a condiment. In the West it is also known as laver.

**Olive oil** A rich Mediterranean cooking oil from the fruit of the olive tree. Used for stir-fries, dressings, condiments, dips for bread, etc. Virgin or extra-virgin olive oil is produced without chemical processing.

**Pressed salad** Sliced or shredded vegetables combined with a marinating agent such as sea salt, umeboshi plums, brown rice vinegar, or shoyu and placed in a pickle press for a few hours. The pressing or pickling retains many of the enzymes and vitamins and makes the vegetables more digestible.

**Quinoa** A tiny high-protein grain native to South America that has a light, nutty flavor. Enjoyed as a main grain and in soups, salads, pasta, and baked goods.

**Rice syrup** A thick sweet syrup made from brown rice used as a concentrated sweetener for desserts, beverages, and special dishes. High in complex carbohydrates, it metabolizes more gradually than simple sugars and helps keep blood sugar levels from rising too rapidly.

**Sea salt** Salt obtained from evaporated seawater and either sun baked or kiln baked. High in trace minerals, it is lower in sodium than ordinary salt and contains no sugar, iodine, or chemical additives. Mild pure white sea salt is recommended in macrobiotic cooking, and grey, yellow, pink, and other lightly colored sea salts or rock salts are avoided as too contractive or hardening to the body.

**Sea vegetables** Edible seaweeds. High in minerals and vitamins, sea vegetables strengthen the blood, contribute flexibility to the circulatory system, and calm and sooth the nerves. They are used daily in macrobiotic cooking in sushi and rice balls, soups, side dishes, and condiments.

**Seitan** High-protein product prepared by cooking wheat gluten with shoyu, kombu, and water. It can be made at home or purchased ready-made at natural foods stores and fashioned into cutlets or grain burgers or added to soups and stews.

**Sesame** Tiny round seeds traditionally eaten in the Far East, Middle East, India, and other parts of the world. Used to make *gomashio*, tahini, sesame butter, sesame oil, and medicinal preparations.

**Shiitake** A mushroom native to the Far East and now grown in North America and throughout the world. The dried variety is used in macrobiotic cooking for soup stocks, vegetable dishes, and medicinal preparations. It is very calming and helps discharge excess animal fat from the body.

**Shiso** A pickled red leaf used to color umeboshi plums and as a condiment. Known in English as beefsteak leaves, it is sometimes spelled *chiso*.

**Shoyu** Traditional, natural soy sauce made from fermented whole soybeans, wheat, and sea salt. Shoyu is best aged naturally for at least a year and not chemically processed. For those on a gluten-free diet, tamari is recommended.

**Soba** Noodles made from buckwheat flour or a combination of buckwheat and whole wheat flour. Soba gives strong, warming energy and may be served in broth, in salads, with vegetables, or lightly chilled in summer.

**Somen** Very thin oriental-style wheat or whole wheat noodles.

**Suribachi** A serrated glazed clay bowl used with a pestle (*surokogi*) for grinding and puréeing foods. It is used for making condiments, spreads, dressings, baby foods, nut butters, and medicinal preparations.

**Sushi** Bite-size pieces of rice wrapped in nori and sliced in rounds. It may contain cucumber, *kampyo* (a gourd), *natto*, umeboshi, avocado, or other ingredients.

**Sweet brown rice** A sweet-tasting variety of glutinous brown rice used to make mochi, ohagi, dumplings, baby foods, brown rice vinegar, and amazake.

**Tahini** A seed butter made by grinding hulled sesame seeds until smooth and creamy.

**Tamari** The liquid poured off during the process of making soybean miso. It is heavier, stronger, and more flavorful than regular shoyu and does not include wheat or gluten. Sold as "original" or "real" tamari, it is used instead of shoyu by those with gluten intolerances or for special dishes.

**Tekka** A condiment made from sautéed *hatcho* miso, sesame oil, burdock, lotus seed, carrots, and ginger root. It is dark brown or black in color and rich in iron and other minerals.

**Tempeh** A soy food made from split soybeans, water, and beneficial bacteria that ferments for several hours. Native to Indonesia, Sri Lanka, and Southeast Asia, it has spread around the world. Rich in protein and vitamin B12, it can be made at home or be obtained ready-made at natural foods stores and supermarkets. It is used in cutlets, sandwiches, soups, stews, and other hardy dishes.

**Tempura** A method of cooking in which seasonal vegetables and other ingredients are coated with batter and deep-fried in vegetable oil. Native to Portugal, it was brought to the Far East and is now used by cooks worldwide.

**Tofu** Soybean curd made from soybeans cooked with *nigari*, a crystallized salt. High in protein, tofu blends well with many other foods and is enjoyed in soups, vegetable dishes, dressings, and frostings.

**Udon** Far Eastern–style noodles made from whole wheat or wheat flour that are lighter than soba. They are served in broth plain or with vegetables, seasoned with shoyu, and garnished with scallions or nori. Leftover udon may be fried.

**Umeboshi plum** A salty pickled plum that stimulates the appetite, aids digestion, and strengthens the blood. Red Shiso leaves impart a bright-red color and natural flavoring to the plums (actually a form of apricot) during pickling. They may be taken whole or in pieces as a condiment, used instead of salt as a seasoning in cooking, be added to rice balls or sushi, or used in medicinal teas.

**Umeboshi paste** A creamy paste made from umeboshi plums. It is used to season corn on the cob and make sauces and other special dishes. It is not as strong as whole umeboshi, which is preferred for medicinal preparations.

**Umeboshi vinegar** A salty, sour vinegar made from umeboshi plums. Diluted with water, it is used in sauces and dressings and as a condiment or seasoning.

**Wakame** A long, thin sea vegetable that cooks up a beautiful translucent green. High in minerals and vitamins, it has a sweet taste and delicate texture and is used in cooking miso soup and a variety of dishes.

**Wheat berries** Wheat kernels in whole form are called wheat berries. They are used to make whole wheat flour and noodles and are cracked or processed into couscous and bulgur. Whole wheat berries are very chewy and are usually cooked together with other grains, beans, or vegetables.

**Wild rice** A wild grass native to the Great Lakes region that grows in water and is harvested by hand. The long, thin dark grains add taste, texture, and flavor to a variety of dishes.

# Macrobiotic Resources

**Planetary Health, Inc.** An educational organization in western Massachusetts directed by Alex Jack, Bettina Zumdick, Edward Esko, and their associates, sponsoring the annual Macrobiotic Summer Conference at Eastover, a holistic resort in Lenox, MA and the Online Winter Macrobiotic Conference. Planetary Health, Inc., the parent nonprofit, also sponsors Amberwaves, a grassroots network to protect rice, wheat, and other grains from genetic engineering, climate change, and other challenges. Amberwaves Press publishes a quarterly journal and books and booklets. Contact: Box 487, Becket MA 01223, 413-623-0012. macrobioticsummerconference.com.

## Macrobiotic Counseling

Personal dietary and way of life sessions are offered by many macrobiotic teachers and counselors in person, by Skype, over the phone, or by written report. While each practitioner has a slightly different approach, they generally include a review of the person's dietary and health history and background, visual diagnosis, specific dietary guidelines, way of life suggestions, and home remedies. Sessions take from about 1 to 1½ hours and cost from $200-$350. Follow up advice is included. To book a consultation with Alex Jack or Bettina Zumdick, please call 413-623-0012 or email Alex **at** shenwa@bcn.net **or** Bettina at Bettinazumdick @verizon.net.

## Books and Literature

### Cookbooks

Kushi, Aveline; Jack, Alex (1985). *Aveline Kushi's Guide to Macrobiotic Cooking for Health, Harmony, and Peace*. Warner Books.

Jack, Alex; Kato, Sachi (2017). *The One Peaceful World Cookbook*: *Over 150 Vegan, Macrobiotic Recipes for Vibrant Health and Happiness,* BenBella.

Tara-Watson, Marlene (2019). *Go Vegan*, Lotus Publications.

Zumdick, Bettina (2012). *Authentic Foods.*

### Diet, Health, and Healing

Kushi, Michio; Jack, Alex (2010). *The Cancer-Prevention Diet*. St. Martin's Press.

Kushi, Michio; Jack, Alex (2002). *The Macrobiotic Path to Total Health*: Ballantine.

Kushi, Michio (2007). *The Do-In Way: Gentle Exercises to Liberate the Body, Mind, and Spirit.* Square One Publications.

Kushi, Michio (2007). *Your Body Never Lies. Square One Publications*

Kushi, Michio; Van Cauwenberge, Marc, M.D. (2014). *Macrobiotic Home Reme-*

*dies*. Square One Publications.

Akizuki, Tatsuichiro, M.D. (1981). *Nagasaki 1945: The First Full-Length Eyewitness Account of the Atomic Bomb Attack on Nagasaki*. Quartet Books.

Andrus, Erik; Elwell, Christian; Rooney, Ben (2017). *The Rice Revolution: Growing Organic Rice in New England*. Amberwaves Press.

*Kushi, Michio (1987). Crime & Diet: The Macrobiotic Approach. Japan Publications.*

Kushi, Michio; Jack, Alex (1985). *Diet for a Strong Heart*. St. Martin's Press.

Kushi, Michio; Kushi, Aveline; Jack, Alex (1985). *Macrobiotic Diet*. Japan Publications, revised 1993.

Porter, Jessica (2011). *The Hip Chick's Guide to Macrobiotics*. Avery Publications,

Waxman, Denny and Susan (2015). *The Complete Macrobiotic Diet*. Pegasus Books.

Yamamoto, Shizuko; McCarthy, Patrick (1979). *Barefoot Shiatsu*. Japan Publications.

## History

Kushi, Michio; Jack, Alex (2013). *The Book of Macrobiotics*. Square One Publications.

Jack, Alex; Esko, Edward, editors (2015*). Remembering Michio*. Kushi Institute.

Kotzsch, Ronald E. (1985). *Macrobiotics: Yesterday and Today*. Japan Publications.

Kushi, Aveline; Jack, Alex (1988). *Aveline: The Life and the Dream of the Woman Behind Macrobiotics Today*. Japan Publications.

Mizuno Namboku (1807); translated by Kushi, Michio; Kushi, Aveline; Jack, Alex (1985). *Food Governs Your Destiny*. Japan Publications, 1992.

Tara, William(1985). *Macrobiotics and Human Behavior*. Japan Publications.

## Philosophy and Science

Kushi, Michio; Jack, Alex (2013). *The Book of Macrobiotics*. Square One Publications.

Butler, Samuel (1870). *Erewhon*. New American Library, 1960.

Esko, Edward (2012). *Yin Yang Primer*. Amberwaves Press.

Esko, Edward; Jack, Alex (2011). *Cool Fusion: A Quantum Solution to Peak Minerals, Nuclear Waste, and Future Metals Shock*. Amberwaves Press.

Esko, Edward; Jack, Alex (2014). *Corking the Nuclear Genie*. Amberwaves Press.

Ferré, Carl, ed. (2013). *Essential Ohsawa: From Food to Health, Happiness to Freedom*. George Ohsawa Macrobiotic Foundation.

Hufeland, Christoph W., M.D. (1796). *Macrobiotics or the Art of Prolonging Life*.

I Ching or Book of Changes (1950). Translated by Richard Wilhelm and Cary F. Baynes. Princeton University Press.

Kervran, Louis (1972). *Biological Transmutations*. 978-0918860651

Kushi, Michio; Jack, Alex (1992). *The Gospel of Peace: Jesus's Teachings of Eternal Truth*. Japan Publications.

Ohsawa, George (1931). *The Unique Principle*: *The Philosophy of Macrobiotics*. George Ohsawa Macrobiotic Foundation, 1973 edition.

Wang, Robin R. (2012). *Yinyang: The Way of Heaven and Earth in Chinese Thought and Culture*. Cambridge University Press.

## Periodicals

*Amberwaves* (2001- ), Becket, Massachusetts

*Macrobiotics Today* (1984- ), Oroville, California

*Das Grosse Leben*, Germany

# About the Authors

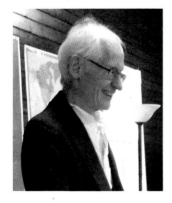

**Alex Jack** is president of Planetary Health and has served as executive director of Kushi Institute and editor-in-chief of *East West Journal*. He has helped introduce macrobiotics to China and Russia and has written many books with Michio and Aveline Kushi, including *The Cancer Prevention Diet*, *Aveline Kushi's Complete Guide to Macrobiotic Cooking*, *The Book of Macrobiotics*, and *One Peaceful World*. He is on the guest faculty of the Kushi Institute of Europe and has presented at the Cardiology Institute in St. Petersburg, the Zen Temple in Beijing, Shakespeare's New Globe Theatre in London, and Rosas Dance Company in Brussels.

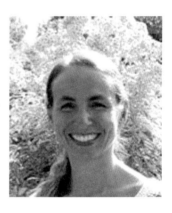

**Bettina Zumdick** is a teacher, counselor, humanitarian, and author who has integrated modern knowledge of the West with the ancient wisdom of the East. With a strong background in Food Science, Dietetics, and Nutrition from Wilhelms University in Muenster, Germany, she has shared her knowledge of food as medicine for over 30 years. Her experience in the fields of holistic health, wellness, and macrobiotics has helped thousands of people to regain and maintain their health and vibrancy. She is the author of *Authentic Foods* and founder of the Culinary Medicine School in Lee, MA. www.culinarymedicineschool.com

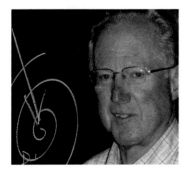

**Edward Esko** is vice president of Planetary Health and has served as associate director of Kushi Institute, executive director of the East West Foundation, and founder of Quantum Rabbit LLC, a new technology company dedicated to a sustainable future. He is the author of *Yin Yang Primer, Rice Field Essays, One Peaceful Universe,* and other books. He is the founder of MacrobioticClassroom: **www.macrobiotic**classroom.com.

# References

[1] *Dietary Guidelines for Americans, 2000*. U.S. Department of Health and Human Services and U.S. Department of Agriculture.

[2] Kushi, Michio; Jack, Alex (2013). *The Book of Macrobiotics: The Universal Way to Health, Happiness, and Peace*. Square One Publications, pp. xii-xvii..

[3] Kushi, Michio; Jack, Alex (2017). *One Peaceful World: Creating a Healthy and Harmonious Mind, Home, and World Community, pp. xii-xvii*. Square One Publications.

[4] Individual studies are listed below.

[5] Kunz, Jeffrey R. M., and Finkel, Asher J., eds. (1987) *The American Medical Association Family Medical Guide*, Random House, p. 27.

[6] Smithsonian Institution Archives. http://siris-archives.si.edu/ipac20/ipac.jsp?profile =all&source.

[7] Kushi, Aveline; Jack, Alex (1985). *Aveline Kushi's Complete Guide to Macrobiotic Cooking*. Warner. ISBN 978-0446386340

[8] Kushi and Jack, *Book of Macrobiotics*, pp. 171-172.

[9] Book of Daniel 1: 8–17. Douay-Rheims American Edition, 1899.

[10] Select Committee on Nutrition and Human Needs, U.S. Senate (1977). *Dietary Goals for the United States*. U.S. Government Printing Office.

[11] Bergan, J. G.; Brown, P. T. "Nutritional Status of 'New' Vegetarians," *Journal of the American Dietetic Association* 76:151-55, 1980.

[12] Hinds, Alison, BSc. "A Short Study of the Macrobiotic Diet." Queen Elizabeth College, University of London, 1985.

[13] Campbell, Ph.D., T. Colin Campbell; Campbell II, Thomas M. (2004, revised 2017), *The China Study*. Benbella Books.

[14] Harmon, Brook E. et al. (2015). "Nutrient Composition and Anti-inflammatory Potential of a Prescribed Macrobiotic Diet," *Nutrition and Cancer*, DOI: 10.1080/01635581.2015.

[15] Smith, Michael, M.D. (2017). "Macrobiotic Diet," Web MD, www.webmd.com. Retrieved March 27, 2017.

[16] Sacks, F. M.; Rosner, Bernard; Kass, Edward H. "Blood Pressure in Vegetarians," *American Journal of Epidemiology* 100:390-98, 1974.

[17] Sacks, F. M. et al. "Plasma Lipids and Lipoproteins in Vegetarians and Controls," *New England Journal of Medicine* 292:1148-51, 1975.

[18] *Healthy People: The Surgeon General's Report on Health Promotion and Disease Prevention*. Government Printing Office, 1979.

[19] Sacks, F. M. et al. "Effects of Ingestion of Meat on Plasma Cholesterol of Vegetarians," *Journal of the American Medical Association* 246:640-44, 1981.

[20] Castelli, William P. "Summary of Lessons from the Framingham Heart Study," Framingham, Mass., September, 1983.

[21] Kushi, Michio; Jack, Alex (1985). *Diet for a Strong Heart*. St. Martin's Press, p. 131. ISBN 978-0312304584

[22] P. Pasanisi et al., "A randomized controlled trial of Mediterranean diet and metformin to prevent age-related diseases in people with metabolic syndrome," *Tumori* 104(2):137-142, Mar-Apr 2018.

[23] Kushi, Michio; Jack, Alex (1985). *Diet for a Strong Heart*. St. Martin's Press, p. 131. 4

[24] H. Kondo et al., "Long-term intake of miso soup decreases nighttime blood pressure in subjects with high-normal blood pressure or stage 1 hypertension," Hypertens Res 42(11):1757-1767, Nov 2019.

[25] Kohler, Jean; Kohler, Marie Ann (1979). *Healing Miracles from Macrobiotics*. Parker Publishing.

[26] Jack and Kushi, *Cancer Prevention Diet*, pp. 403–404.

[27] Dobic, Milenka (2000). *My Beautiful Life*. Avery Publishing.

[28] Benedict, Dirk (1991). Confessions of a Kamikaze Cowboy. Avery.

[29] Nussbaum, Elaine (1992). *Recovery: From Cancer to Health Through Macrobiotics*. Japan Publications.

[30] Kushi and Jack, *The Cancer Prevention Diet*, pp. 430–431. St. Martin's Press.

[31] *One Peaceful World Journal*, #6 August 1990.

[32] Satillaro, Anthony J., M.D.; Monte, Tom (1982). *Recalled by Life: The Story of My Recovery from Cancer*, Houghton-Mifflin, 1982.

[33] Kushi and Jack, *Cancer-Prevention Diet*, pp. 313–314. *One Peaceful World Journal* #5, Spring, 1991.

[34] Kushi and Jack, *Cancer-Prevention Diet*, p. 351.

[35] Brown, Virginia, R.N.; Stayman, Susan (1982). Macrobiotic Miracle: How a Vermont Family Overcame Cancer. Japan Publications.

[36] The East West Foundation and Ann Fawcett (1992). *Cancer-Free: 30 Who Triumphed Over Cancer Naturally*. Japan Publications..

[37] Geismar, Erin, "Montauk Man Still Cancer-Free After 6 Years," *East Hampton Press*, March 2, 2010.

[38] NIH Best Cases Study. University of South Carolina, Prevention Research Center, 2002.

[39] Minutes of the Fifth Meeting, Cancer Advisory Panel for Complementary and Alternative Medicine (CAPCAM), Bethesda, Maryland, February 25, 2002; Ralph Moss, Ph.D., "The Olive Branch Bears Fruit," *The Moss Reports*, February 27, 2002. www.cancerdecisions. com/022702.html

[40] Macrobiotic Research Project," Jane Teas, Ph.D., principal investigator; Joan Cunningham, Ph.D., co-principal investigator, sponsored by the Centers for Disease Control, October 2000 to September 2002, University of South Carolina, Prevention Research Center, School of Public Health, Charleston, S.C. www.macro-biotics.sph.sc.edu/project.htm

[41] "Nutrition and Special Diet: Macrobiotics," M.D. Anderson Cancer Center, the University of Texas,www.mdanderson.org/depart ments/cime, 2003-2006.

[42] B. R. Goldin et al. "Effect of Diet on Excretion of Estrogens in Pre- and Postmenopausal Incidence of Breast Cancer in Vegetarian Women," *Cancer Research* 41:3771-73, 1981.

[43] Teas, J; Harbison, M. L.; Gelman, R.S. (1984). "Dietary Seaweed [*Laminaria*] and Mammary Carcinogenesis in Rats, Cancer Research 44:2758-61.

[44] Yamamoto; Ichiro; et al. (1987). "The Effect of Dietary Seaweeds on 7,12-Dimethyl-Benz[a]Anthracene-Induced Mammary Tumorigenesis in Rats," *Cancer Letters* 35:109–18.

[45] Berrino, Franco et al. "Reducing Bioavailable Sex Hormones through a Comprehensive Change in Diet: the Diet and Androgens (DIANA) Randomized Trial," *Cancer Epidemiology, Biomarkers, & Prevention* 10: 25-33, January 2001.

[46] Allen, N.E. et al. "The associations of diet with serum insulin-like growth factor I and its main bind-ing proteins in 292 women meat-eaters, vegetarians, and vegans. *Cancer Epidemiol Biomarkers Prev.* 2002;11(11):1441-1448.

[47] Nkondjock, A. et al. "Diet Quality and BRCA-associated breast cancer risk," Breast Cancer Res Treat. 2007 Jul;103(3):361-9. 84 Nkondjock A. et al., "Diet, lifestyle and BRCA-related breast cancer risk among French-Canadians," *Breast Cancer Res Treat.* 2006 Aug;98(3):285-94. Ghadirian P., et al., "Breast cancer risk in relation to the joint effect of BRCA mutations and diet diversity," *Breast Cancer Res Treat.* 2009 Sep;117(2):417-22.

[48]Jernstrom, H. et al., "Breast-feeding and the risk of breast cancer in BRCA1 and BRCA2 mutation carriers," *Journal National Cancer Institute*, 2004;96(14):1094-1098.

13. Cho E, Spiegelman D, Hunter DJ, et al. Premenopausal fat intake and risk of breast cancer. *J Natl Cancer Inst.* 95:1079-85, 2003.

14. "High-Fat Dairy Products Linked to Poorer Breast Cancer Survival," Kaiser Permanente, Press Re-lease, March 14, 2013.

[51] Jack, Alex et al. (2013*). Nutrition vs. Surgery: The Breast Cancer Controversy*, p. 3–10. Amberwaves Press.

[52] Barillari, J. et al. "Kaiware Daikon (*Raphanus sativus L.*) extract: a naturally multipotent chemopre-ventive agent," *J Agric Food Chem.* 2008 Sep 10;56(17):7823-30.

[53] Ollberding, N.J. et al. "Legume, soy, tofu, and isoflavone intake and endometrial cancer risk in postmenopausal women in the multiethnic cohort study," *J Natl Cancer Inst* 2012 Jan4;104(1):67-76.

[54] A. Nakamura et al. "Genistein inhibits cell invasion and motility by inducing cell differentiation in murine osteosarcoma cell line LM8, *BMC Cell Biol.* 2012 Sep 26;13:24.

[55] Carter, James P. et al. "Hypothesis: Dietary Management May Improve Survival from Nutritionally Linked Cancers Based on Analysis of Representative Cases," *Journal of the American College of Nutrition* 12:209-226, 1993.

[56] Ibid.

[57] Saxe, G.A. et al. "Potential Attenuation of Disease Progression in Recurrent Prostate Cancer with Plant-Based Diet and Stress Reduction," *Integr Cancer Ther* 5(3)206-13, 2006.

[58] Hirayama, T. "Relationship of Soybean Paste Soup Intake to Gastric Cancer Risk," *Nutrition and Cancer* 3: 223–33.

[59] Chihara, G. et al. "Fractionation and Purification of the Polysaccharides with Marked Antitumor Activity, Especially Lentinan, from *Lentinus edodes* (Berk.) Sing. (An Edible Mushroom), *Cancer Research* 30: 2776–81.

[60] "Complementary and Alternative Therapies, American Cancer Society Internet Site, 1997; "Alternative and Complementary Therapies," *Cancer* 77(6), 1996.

[61] "Guide for Nutrition and Physical Activity for Cancer Survivors," *CA: A Cancer Journal for Clinicians*, Sept.-Oct. 2003.

[62] American Cancer Society guidelines on nutrition and physical activity for cancer prevention (2012), Lawrence H. Kushi ScD. CA: *A Cancer Journal for Clinicians* Volume 62, Issue 1 January/February 2012. Pages 30–67.

[63] Sadovsky, Richard. "Complementary and Alternative Medical Therapies for Cancer," *American Family Physician*, May 1, 2003.

[64] S. M. Zick et al., "Pros and Cons of Dietary Strategies Popular Among Cancer Patients," *Oncology* 15;32(11);542-547, Nov 2018.

[65] American Cancer Society (2012), op cit.

[66] "Patients with Kaposi Sarcoma Who Opt for No Treatment," Letter. *Lancet*, July 1985.

[67] Kushi, Michio; Jack (1995). *AIDS and Beyond: Dietary and Lifestyle Guidelnes for New Viral and Bacterial Disease.* One Peaceful World Press. (1997) *Humanity at the Crossroads.* One Peaceful Word Press. (2003) *Macrobiotic Path to Total Health.*

[68] "Umeboshi Have H1N1 Suppressant," *Japan Times,* June 3, 2010.

[69] Hafstraim, I. et al. "A Vegan Diet Free of Gluten Improves the Symptoms of Rheumatoid Arthritis," *Rheumatology* 40(10):1175-79, 2001.

[70] McDougall, John. "Diet: The Only Real Hope for Arthritis," *The McDougall Newsletter*, May/June, 1998.

[71] Childers, N. F.; Margoles, M. S. "An Apparent Relation of Nightshades (Solanaceae) to Arthritis," *Journal of Neurological and Orthopedic Medical Surgery* 12:227-231, 1993.

[72] Campbell, Don (1997). *The Mozart Effect.* Avon Books.

[73] Harvey, Judy. "Overcoming Autism with Diet," *One Peaceful World Journal* 29:1, Winter 1997.

[74] Anonymous. *Macrobiotic Recovery from Autism,* Planetary Health/Amberwaves, 2014.

[75] Knivsber, A. M. et al. "Reports on Dietary Intervention in Autistic Disorders," *Nutri Neurosci* (4)1:25-37, 2001. A. M. Knivsber et al., "A Randomized Study of Dietary Intervention in Autistic Syndrome," *Nutr Neurosci* 5(4):251-61, 2002.

[76] Jack, Alex. "The Origin of Celiac," *Amberwaves Journal*, Spring 2014.

[77] Ventura, Valerie. "A Comparative Study of the Meals Provided for Pre-School Children by Two Day Nurseries," Department of Nutrition, Queen Elizabeth College, 1980.

[78] Shull, M. W. et al. "Velocities of Growth in Vegetarian Preschool Children," *Pediatrics* 60:410-17, 1977.

[79] Dwyer, J. T. et al. "Mental Age and I.Q. of Predominantly Vegetarian Children," *Journal of the American Dietetic Association* 76:142-47, 1980.

[80] Esko, Edward; Jack, Alex; and Harper, Virginia. *Crohn's and Colitis: The Macrobiotic Approach,* Amberwaves Press, 2016.

[81] Bhjumisawasdi, J. et al. "The Self-Reliant System for Alternative Care of Diabetes Mellitus Patients—Experience Macrobiotic Management in Trad Province," *Journal of the Medical Association of Thailand* 89(12):2104-15, 2006.

[82] Porrata, Carmen, M.D., PhD., et al. "Ma-Pi 2 Macrobiotic Diet Intervention in Adults with Type 2 Diabetes Mellitus," *MEDICC Review*, Fall 2009, 11(4):29-35.

[83] Hu, Emily A. et al. "White rice consumption and risk of type 2 diabetes: meta-analysis and systematic review, *BMJ* 2012; 344.

[84] Lerman, Robert H., M.D., Ph.D. "The Macrobiotic Diet in Chronic Disease," *Nutri Clin Prac* December 2010; 25(6):621-626.

[85] D. Papamichou et al., "Dietary patterns and management of type 2 diabetes: A systematic review of randomized clinical trials," *Nutri Metab Cardiovasc Dis* 29(5):531-543, June 2019.

[86] Jack, Alex; Esko, Edward (2014). *Ebola & Diet.* Planetary Health, Inc., Michio Kushi with the Kushi Institute Research and Faculty Committee, *Ebola Relief and Prevetion: Dieary Recommendations and Proposals.* Kushi Institute, 2014. www.ebolaanddiet.com

[87] Rogers, Sherry A. M.D. "From HEAL's Advisory Board: The Cure Is in the Kitchen—One Case History," *The Human Ecologist*, Fall 1990, pp. 19-21.

[88] Rogers, Sherry A., M.D. "Improvement in Chemical Sensitivity with the Macrobiotic Diet," *Journal of Applied Nutrition* 48: 85-92, 1996.

[89] Lieff, Jonathan et al. (1987). "Study Results of Dietary Change in Shattuck Hospital Geropsychiatric Wards, 5 North and 6 North," in Michio Kushi, *Crime and Diet*, pp. 229-34.

[90] Green, Peter (2010). *Celiac Disease: A Hidden Epidemic.* William Morrow. ISBN 978-0060766948.

[91] Thomas, Katya. "I Love Gluten," *Amberwaves Journal*, Autumn 2012.

[92] Iglehart, Tom (1987). "The Shattuck Model: Macrobiotics in an Institution," in Michio Kushi et al., *Crime and Diet*. Japan Publications, 1987, pp. 203-29. ISBN 978-0870406829.

[93] Armelin, Cecilia. "Wholefood Diet," National Children's Hospital, Dublin, Ireland, 1989.

[94] C. Ekmekcioglu, "Nutrition and longevity—From mechanisms to uncertainties," *Crit Rev Food Sci Nutr* 21:1-20, Oct 2019.

[95] Wetzel, Miriam S. et al. "Courses Involving Complementary and Alternative Medicine at U.S. Medical Schools." *Journal of the American Medical Association* 280:784-87, 1998.

[96] "Most medical schools offer courses in alternative medicine." Vox.com, July 8, 2015.

[97] Briscoe, David; Mahoney-Briscoe, Charlotte (1989). *A Personal Peace: Macrobiotic Reflections on Mental and Emotional Recovery: Macrobiotic Reflections on Mental and Emotional Recovery.* Japan Publications..

[98] Harnish, Stephen, M.D. (1989). "On My Awakening to the Macrobiotic Way," *Doctors Look at Macrobiotics*. Japan Publications. ISBN 978-0870406867.

[99] Blanc, Bernard H.; Hertel, Hans U. "Influence on Man: Comparative Study About Food Prepared Conventionally and in the Microwave Oven," *Raum & Zeit*, 3(2): 1992.

[100] Farrell, H.V. (1988). "PMS Is Not PMS," *Doctors Look at Macrobiotics*, pp. 177-91.

[101] Sand I. Katz et al., "Randomized-controlled trial of a modified Mediterranean dietary program for multiple sclerosis: A pilot study," *Multi Scler Relat Disord* 24;36:101403, Sep 2019.

[102] Akizuki, Tatsuichiro, M.D. *Nagasaki 1945* (1980). Quartet Books, 1981. Akizuki, Tatsuichiro, M.D., "How We Survived Nagasaki," *East West Journal*, December 1980.

[103] Furo, Hiroko, Ph.D. "Dietary Practices of Hiroshima/Nagasaki Atomic Bomb Survivors," Illinois Wesleyan University, 2006.

[104] Skoryna, S.C. et al. "Studies on Inhibition of Intestinal Absorption of Radioactive Strontium," *Canadian Medical Association Journal* 91: 285-88, 1964.

[105] "Miso Shows Promise as Treatment for Radiation," *Japan Times,* September 27, 1988.

[106] Jack, Alex. "Soviets Embrace Macrobiotics," *One Peaceful World* 6:1 Autumn/Winter, 1990.

[107] "Effects of agar (kanten) diet on obese patients with impaired glucose tolerance and type 2 diabetes," *Diabetes, Obesity, and Metabolism*, 7(1):40–46, 2005.

[108] Ikeda, Y. et al. "Intake of Fermented Soybeans, Natto, Is Associated with Reduced Bone Loss in Postmenopausal Women: Japanese Population-Based Osteoporosis (JPOS) Study," *J Nutri* 136(5):1323-8, 2006.

[109] Cardini, F.; Weixin, H. "Moxibustion for correction of breech presentation: a randomized controlled trial," *JAMA.* 1998 Nov 11;280(18):1580-4.

[110] Coyle, M. E. et al. "Cephalic version by moxibustion for breech presentation,"

*Cochrane Database Syst Rev.* 2012 May 16;(5):CD003928.

[111] Amir, N. et al. "Efficacy comparison between Chinese medicine's labor inducement methods and conventional methods customary in hospitals," *Harefuah.* 2015 Jan;154(1):47-51, 67, 66.

[112] Jack, Alex; Jack, Gale (2006). *Chewing Made Easy: 42 Benefits, Tips, and Techniques.* Macrobiotic Path.

[113] "The Veggie Baseball Team," *Parade Magazine*, April 15, 1984.

[114] Walsh, Michael. "Sounds of Silence," *Time*, June 24, 2001.

[115] "Bushmen," NationalGeographic.com, January 2000.

[116] Richards, M.P. "A Brief Review of the Archaeological Evidence for Palaeolithic and Neolithic Subsistence," *Eur J Clin Nutri* 2002 Dec;56(12):1262-78.

[117] Wrangham, Richard (2009). *Catching Fire: How Cooking Made Us Human.* Basic Books 2009.

[118] "Diet likely changed game for some hominids 3.5 million years ago," ScienceDaily.com, June 13, 2013. *Proceedings of the National Academy of Sciences*, June 3, 2013.

[119] Ferran Estebaranz, et al. "Buccal dental microwear analyses support greater specialization in consumption of hard foodstuffs for *Australopithecus anamensis.*" *Journal of Anthropological Sciences*, 2012; 90: 1-24.

[120] Mercader, Julio, "Mozambican Grass Seed Consumption During the Middle Stone Age," *Science* 326:Dec. 18, 2009. www.sciencemag.org.

[121] Fairservis, Walter Ashlin (1975). *The Threshold of Civilization: An Experiment in Prehistory.* Charles Scribner's Sons.

[122] "The Stone Age baker: Cavemen 'ate bread, not just meat.'" *Daily Mail Reporter*, October 19, 2010.

[123] *Amberwaves Journal* 2001-2017.

[124] Jack, Alex (2000). *Imagine a World Without Monarch Butterflies: Awakening to the Hazards of Genetically Altered Foods*, foreword by Congressman Dennis J. Kucinich. One Peaceful World Press.

[125] Cummins, Joseph (2001). "The First Independent Study of Genetically Engineered LibertyLink Rice," www.amberwaves.org.

[126] Schoenthaler, S., Ph.D. "The Effect of Sugar on the Treatment and Control of Antisocial Behavior," *International Journal of Biosocial Research* 3(1):1-9, 1982.

[127] Seaker, Meg. "Fighting Crime with Diet: Report from a Portuguese Prison," *East West Journal*, July, 1982, pp. 26-34.

[128] Jack, Alex (2002). *Sex, Lies, and GMOs*, Amberwaves Press.

[129] Kushi and Jack, *One Peaceful World*, pp. 28–31.

[130] Kushi and Jack, *One Peaceful World*, pp. 38–39.

[131] "Bringing Brown Rice and Peace to Syria," *Amberwaves Journal*, Summer 2012.

[132] Kushi and Jack, *One Peaceful World*, pp. 75–77.

[133] Jack, Alex. "Nutrition Under Siege," *One Peaceful World Journal* 34:1, 7–9, 1998.

[134] *Livestock's Long Shadow*, UN Food & Agricultural Organization, 2006.

[135] Eishel, Gidon; Martin Pamela. "Study: vegan diets healthier for planet, people than meat diets," *Earth Interactions*, April 2006.

[136] Loladze, I (2014). "Hidden shift of the ionome of plants exposed to elevated CO2 depletes minerals at the base of human nutrition." elife. 2014 3:e02245
http://www.researchgate.net/profile/Irakli_Loladze

[137] "Mobile Phones Could Lead to Bee Decline, *The Ecologist*, April 2007.

[138] "Cell Phones," National Toxicology Program, last modified Sep. 13, 2016,
http://ntp.niehs.nih.gov/results/areas/cellphones/. "Cell Phone Radiation Boos Cancer Rates in Animals; $25 Million NTP Study Finds Brain Tumors," *Microwave News*, May 25, 2016. "ACS Responds to New Study Linking Cell Phone Radiation to Cancer," American Cancer Society, May 2017, http://pressroomcancer.org/NTP2016.

[139] Kervran, Louis C. (1972). *Biological Transmutations*, Swan House.

[140] Kushi, Michio; Esko, Edward (1994). *The Philosopher's Stone.* One Peaceful World Press.

[141] Goldfein, Solomon. "Energy Development from Elemental Transmutations in Biological Systems," Report 2247, Ft. Belvoir, Va.: U.S. Army Mobility Equipment Research and Development Command, 1978.

[142] Esko, Edward; Jack, Alex (2011). *Cool Fusion: A Quantum Solution to Peak Minerals, Nuclear Waste and Future Metal Shock*. Amberwaves Press.

[143] Falchi et al. The new world atlas of artificial night sky brightness," *Sci. Adv.* 2016;2.

[144] Jack, Alex. "A Dark Starless World," *Amberwaves Journal,* Autumn 2016.

[145] Kushi and Jack, *Book of Macrobiotics*, p. 4.

Made in the USA
Columbia, SC
26 May 2021

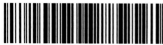
38149384R00064